Less Stress, Better Health

Less Stress, Better Health

How Stress Impacts Your Health and What You Can Do About It

Dr. Fran Addeo

Cover design by Doug Crowe

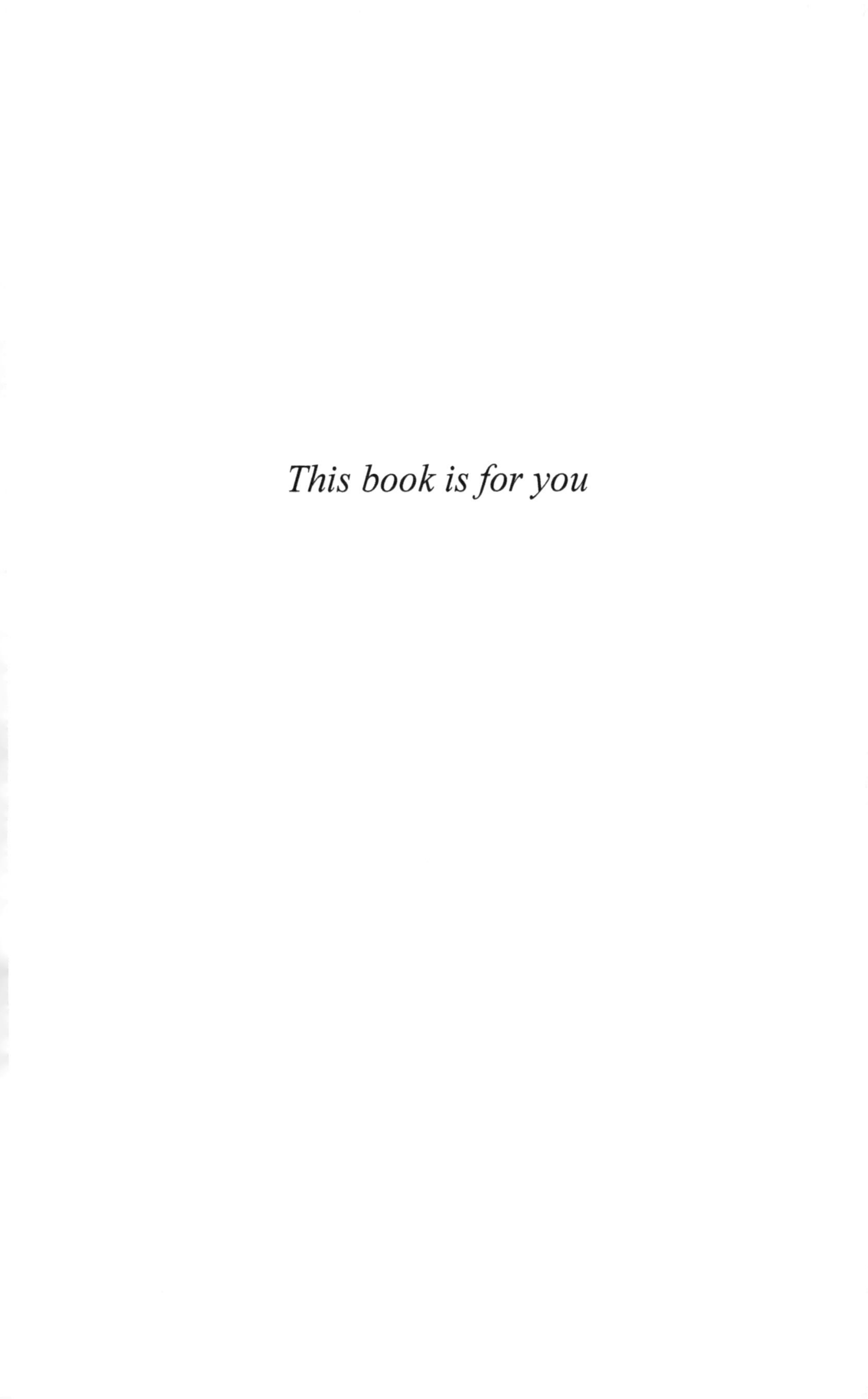

This book is for you

Table of Contents

Preface xiii

Introduction: Stress is the Problem xvii

How to Use This Book xxi

Part I – Emotional Stress

Chapter 1: The Stress Response 3
Fight-or-Flight 4
Rest and Digest 5
The Dopamine Dilemma 6

Chapter 2: How the Brain and Body Work Together . . 9
The Spinal Cord 10
The Vagus Nerve 10

Chapter 3: Improving Vagal Tone 12
Singing and Sound-Based Techniques 12
The Role of Laughter 13

Chapter 4: Calming the Body 16
Meditation 17
Mindfulness 17
Breathing Practices 19

Chapter 5: Daily Mindfulness Techniques 23

Mindful Hydration 24

Silent Walking 24

The Healing Power of Nature 25

Chapter 6: The Human Mind is a Mystery 28

The Conscious Mind 29

The Subconscious Mind 29

Chapter 7: Reprogramming Thought Patterns 31

Affirmations 32

Neuroplasticity 32

Challenge yourself 33

Chapter 8: Hypnosis 38

Helped Mayo Clinic 39

Slowing Down Brain Waves 39

Autogenic Training 40

Chapter 9: The HeartMath Institute 44

A HeartMath Exercise 45

Promoting Global Coherence 46

Chapter 10: Emotional Triggers 48

Scan, Sense, Soothe 48

Name it to Tame it 49

Chapter 11: Processing Emotions 51

Crying 52

Venting 53

Shake It Off 55

Emotional Freedom Technique (EFT) 56

Chapter 12: Resilience and Reframing 59

Who's to Say? 60

Living the Dream 61

Gratitude 62

Chapter 13: When to Seek Help 63

The Top-Down Approach 64

Other Brain-Based Techniques 64

How to Find a Therapist 68

Part II – Chemical Stress

Chapter 14: Chemicals in Our Food 73

Fear Not 73

Made in the USA 74

SAD DAD 75

Chapter 15: The Food Industry 77

Ultra-Processed Foods (UPFs) 79

Not All Processed Foods Are Bad 80

Chapter 16: Scientific Studies 83

Think for Yourself 84

Fatty Acids, Seed Oils 85

Choosing a Diet 89

Chapter 17: What's in Your Kitchen? 93

Food as Fuel 95

The 80/20 Rule 97

Eating Healthy on a Budget 97

Chapter 18: It's Never Too Late 101
Transmutation? 102
Rest and Digest 103
Giving Thanks 103

Chapter 19: Our Digestive Tube 105
Our Second Brain 106
Gut-Brain Axis 107
Our Gut Bacteria 109
Happy Liver Day! 112

Chapter 20: Environmental Toxins 115
Constitution vs. Condition 117
Hormones 121
Dirty Dozen, Clean Fifteen 127

Chapter 21: Inflammation 131
How to Reduce Inflammation. 132
Oxidative Stress 133

Chapter 22: A Pill for Every ill 136
Ask Your Doctor 137
Polypharmacy 138
Deprescribing – an Emerging Specialty? 139

Chapter 23: The Flexner Report 143
Integrative Medicine .144

Part III – Physical Stress

Chapter 24: Inside Information .149
Bones Make Joints 149
Ligaments as Springs 149
Muscles and Tendons 150

Chapter 25: Our Back Bone 152
Cartilage Discs 152
Hydration 153
Arthritis 156

Chapter 26: Low Back Pain 158
Failed Back Surgery 159
Goobie Doobie 160

Chapter 27: Ergonomics 162
Posture 162
Sitting 164
Text Neck 165

Chapter 28: Exercise 169
Wake-up Stretch Routine 170
Benefits of Walking 174
Building and Maintaining Muscle Strength 176

Chapter 29: Recovery after Exercise 180
A Good Night's Sleep 181
The Glymphatic System 182
Leave the Day Behind 183

Chapter 30: Preventing Injuries 186
Household Tasks 187
Lifting 187

Chapter 31: Self-Care for Minor Injuries 190
No Heat for Injuries 191
Heat for Arthritis? 192

Chapter 32: What About Chiropractic? 194
Not true! 195
Chiropractic Philosophy 197
A Better Way to Heal 201

Conclusion 209

Acknowledgments 211

Bibliography 213

References 215

Preface

Once upon a time — in what now seems like a past life — I was suffering extreme physical and emotional pain after a car accident.

I didn't know it at the time, but when we feel pain, the limbic system in the brain creates emotions, which explains the fear, worry, and anxiety I was feeling.

In an attempt to relieve my neck and lower back pain, my orthopedic surgeon prescribed drug after drug, but none of them worked. After two years, as the pain shooting down my leg got worse and worse, he said I needed back surgery. At 28 years old, I was a physical and emotional wreck.

> *We're never given a problem*
> *without a gift in its hand.*
> —Richard Bach

During those dark nights of my soul, I was working as a feature writer for the *Fort Lauderdale News*. As fate or destiny would have it, I was given an assignment by my editor to interview and write a story about Dr. Wayne Dyer for *The Fort Lauderdale Magazine*.

Wayne's bestselling book, *Your Erroneous Zones*, explained how to break free from negative emotions by changing your thoughts. As a psychologist who wanted to help people, Wayne could tell I needed help. He gave me two suggestions:

1. Go see his chiropractor.
2. Quit my job at the newspaper and write a book.

Going to a chiropractor seemed like a strange thing to do, but he gave me the name of his chiropractor and I called to make an appointment.

As the chiropractor explained, the adjustment would reduce interference to the nerves exiting from between the bones of my spine. After my first adjustment, I was pleasantly surprised because I felt some immediate relief. It took two or three visits for the pain to subside to the point that I was able to get back to taking walks on the beach.

Before long, I quit my job at the newspaper and began my healing journey. Eventually, I looked into becoming a chiropractor, but when I found out how long it would take and how much it would cost, I enrolled in massage therapy school instead.

By the time I graduated from massage therapy school, I had already begun taking the first of many college courses I would need to get into chiropractic college.

Going back to college for courses — including chemistry and physics and the math required for them — was challenging, but I did it. At the age of 37, I enrolled in Life Chiropractic College in Marietta, Georgia, and began almost four years of intense study, including dissecting cadavers. Yuck!

Becoming a chiropractor was a big undertaking and resulted in a huge student loan, but after studying day and night for years, in 1992, at the age of 41, I graduated as a Doctor of Chiropractic.

I've been a chiropractor for more than 30 years. I've helped thousands of patients, and I've learned a lot about health and healing. As I tell my patients, "Health is my hobby." I hope health becomes yours too – because, as a massage therapist had printed on his business card,

"The best thing to save for old age is yourself."

Introduction

Stress is the Problem

Sixty percent of Americans suffer from at least one chronic disease made worse by stress, including heart disease, cancer, diabetes, obesity, and arthritis.

Although stress may not be the primary reason for a patient visit, up to 90 percent of all doctor visits are stress-related. Stress affects every aspect of our life and plays an important role in health and well-being.

We often think of stress in terms of emotional stress, but emotional, chemical, and physical stress are interconnected. They create a biological feedback loop, keeping us stuck in a vicious cycle that destroys our health and sense of well-being.

The following is a brief example of how these three types of stress feed each other and why all three types of stress need to be addressed.

- Emotional stress causes chemical stress by triggering the release of stress hormones such as adrenaline and cortisol. These raise the heart rate and blood pressure and cause inflammation, which leads to physical stress — including pain.

- Physical stress, such as pain or lack of sleep, causes emotional stress, which then triggers the release of stress hormones that leads to chemical stress.

- Chemical stress leads to physical stress, which then triggers emotional stress.

This book is divided into three main sections with each section providing insight, information, helpful tips, and inspiration for reducing and managing all three types of stress. Understanding how these three types of stress keep us stuck in a negative feedback loop and learning simple things we can do to reduce all three types of stress gives us the power to break the cycle.

Emotional Stress

In Part One, you will become aware of the internal sources of emotional stress and how they affect the physiology of the body. Practical, easy-to-learn tools such as breathwork, mindfulness, vagal tone regulation, and emotion-processing techniques will be explained in easy-to-understand terms.

Emotional stress hormones can lead to poor sleep, chronic tension, mood instability, and burnout. The information in this section will help regulate your body's reaction to stress through simple, natural tools. You will be guided on a journey from reacting to challenges in an unconscious way to emotional mastery. By stabilizing the mind, we can interrupt our body's physical reaction to stress and become better able to handle the challenges of life.

Chemical Stress

In Part Two, we will confront the external sources of stress, including chemicals in our food, our environment, and pharmaceutical overload. This section provides information you need to make informed decisions that will help you reclaim your chemical balance. It exposes systemic failures in public health and will help you face the truth, renew control, and do what it takes to reduce chemical stress on your body.

Physical Stress

Part Three is about improving structure and conditioning of our physical body. Information to build strength, prevent injuries, and improve and maintain alignment will help you maximize your health potential.

As you reconnect with your body as a source of vitality rather than pain and limitation, you will become more resilient and motivated to continue on the path to becoming a new and better version of yourself.

How to Use This Book

You can read this book from beginning to end, or use it as a manual by looking over the table of contents and choosing the chapters you want to read. Many different techniques are presented and it may seem like a lot to absorb. You may want to read through it quickly, try one or two ideas, and then go back and read it again more slowly. Becoming familiar with the contents will help you use this book as a reference guide for managing stress.

The three types of stress are interconnected, so you can begin by addressing any one of them.

- Reducing emotional stress will reduce the level of stress hormones in your body, lessening chemical and physical stress, including physical pain and discomfort.

- Reducing chemical stress that causes pain and inflammation will reduce physical stress that leads to emotional stress.

- Reducing physical stress makes it easier to manage emotional stress, leading to less chemical stress.

We are all different, and what works for one person might not work for another. By using the techniques in this book that appeal to you, you will have the tools to shift your body out of stress mode and back into balance, even in the middle of daily chaos.

Thank you for being here with me on this journey to making the rest of your life the best of your life. Let's get started.

Part I

Emotional Stress

Chronic emotional stress from the challenges of everyday life floods the body with stress hormones that disrupt nearly every area of health, including sleep, digestion, immunity, heart health, and mood.

This section provides information to help you master your body's automatic stress response.

Emotional stress feeds chemical and physical stress, keeping you stuck in a negative feedback loop. The strategies in this section calm the nervous system and break that harmful cycle.

Learning how to regulate the body's automatic stress response is a skill that promotes vitality, balance, and a deep sense of well-being. As the conscious mind gains control over automatic stress responses, inner peace emerges, allowing you to live with greater clarity and connection to your true nature.

Chapter One

The Stress Response

You have power over your mind, not outside events.
Realize this, and you will find strength.

—Marcus Aurelius

Learning to manage our emotions is the most important thing we can do to improve our health. According to the Mayo Clinic and other health experts, emotional stress can lead to chronic conditions such as:

- Diabetes

- Digestive problems

- Heart disease

- Strokes

- Dementia

Fight-or-Flight

Fight-or-flight is an automatic reflex that helped early humans survive danger when living in the wild. It describes the physical changes that happen to our body when our senses detect danger. When we see, hear, smell, taste, or feel danger, our adrenal glands automatically respond by releasing stress hormones. These hormones, including adrenaline and cortisol, are chemical messengers that send signals throughout our body. They provide a burst of energy to help us either fight or flee from danger.

Fight-or-flight, also known as the *sympathetic mode,* puts us in survival mode. When we go into fight-or-flight, the following things happen to our body:

- Blood leaves the digestive system and goes to muscles, which provides extra strength to fight or run.

- Heart rate increases, pumping more oxygen to the muscles.

- Glucose is released into the bloodstream for energy.

False Alarms

Even if there is no threat of physical danger, emotions such as fear, anger, worry, and anxiety also trigger fight-or-flight. Our thoughts stimulate the release of stress hormones. Some everyday situations that give rise to emotions that trigger fight-or-flight include:

- Financial stress

- Physical pain

- Conflict with a family member or friend

- Being stuck in traffic

Maintaining a Balance

Not all stress is bad. There are situations in life where a surge of energy helps us:

- Achieve our goals

- Participate in an athletic event

- Give a good public performance

Most people do not know how to manage stress. They live their lives in a constant state of fight-or-flight which can harm their health. Learning to manage stress — and maintaining a balance between "fight-or-flight and "rest and digest" is the key to a balanced life.

Rest and Digest

Rest and digest, also known as the *parasympathetic* mode, is the opposite of fight or flight. Spending time in rest-and-digest lowers stress hormones, improves digestion, helps us sleep better, and increases *happy hormones*. Happy hormones include the following:

- **Serotonin** creates a long-lasting feeling of happiness or well-being.

- **Oxytocin** creates a feeling of love when bonding with a person or playing with a pet.

- **Endorphins** produced by the body during exercise provide a sense of well-being.

- **Dopamine** gives a temporary sense of pleasure when completing a task, eating high-sugar food, using caffeine, nicotine, cocaine, having sex, gaming, or getting a "like" on social media posts.

The Dopamine Dilemma

As part of the brain's reward system, dopamine inspires us to seek pleasure and avoid pain. The temporary pleasure we get from dopamine is more about the anticipation and pursuit of pleasure than actual satisfaction. Dopamine released during a pleasurable activity doesn't necessarily lead to happiness because it leaves us wanting more.

This feel-good hormone has been linked to addiction, which is why social media, video games, and other activities can become addictive. In today's world of constant notifications and instant entertainment, the frequent release of dopamine can lead to fatigue and anxiety, as overstimulation wears down our dopamine receptors. Constant connectivity can become a serious problem, but there are things we can do to break this cycle.

What You Can Do

- Set time limits and intentions before scrolling.

- Turn off notifications for news and media.

- Take digital detox breaks.

Doomscrolling

While we may want to stay informed, excessive scrolling through our phones or computers and reading bad news can trigger the release of stress hormones. Doomscrolling can lessen our ability to focus on things we can control. This can leave us feeling sad, anxious, and overwhelmed.

Instead of doom scrolling, it would be better to watch something funny, look at family photos, or read uplifting stories. We need to become mindful of the dangers of dopamine addiction, but some scientists say we can also become addicted to stress hormones!

Addicted to Stress Hormones?

"Adrenaline junkies" is a term used to describe people who engage in high-intensity activities such as sky diving, motocross, starting fights, or other exciting — but potentially dangerous — activities. The rush of adrenaline into their bloodstream provides a temporary burst of energy and alertness. This can feel exhilarating and leave them wanting more.

Craving the release of stress hormones or dopamine is not really considered to be an addiction, since it doesn't involve an external substance, but it is important to recognize that we can become dependent upon stress hormones.

Some successful people who thrive under pressure may look at rest and relaxation as laziness or lack of motivation. This can lead to spending too much time in fight-or-flight. Recognizing this danger can help maintain a healthy balance. Becoming dependent upon stress hormones circulating in the blood can cause inflammation and lead to the development of chronic diseases.

The Takeaway

The first step in learning to manage emotions is understanding your body's automatic response to stress. This will help you recognize what's happening in your body when you feel anxiety, tension, and other disturbing emotions. As you become aware of your body's response to emotions, you can use simple tools to regulate your nervous system, stabilize your mind, and improve your health and sense of well-being.

The following chapter explains how the nervous system controls the body. Understanding how your body and brain work together empowers you to recognize and control stress before it controls you.

Chapter Two

How the Brain and Body Work Together

Our brain and nervous system control every function of the body. It can be thought of as the electrical system of the body. Understanding how our control center works can help us identify ways to manage our emotional stress.

The Brain Has Three Main Parts

- **The Reptilian Brain:** Located at the bottom back area of our skull, this part of the brain controls automatic processes that keep us alive, such as breathing, heartbeat, body temperature, and digestion. It plays a vital role in survival and instinct and is closely associated with the limbic system.

- **The Limbic System:** Located deep within the brain, this system regulates emotions. It includes the amygdala, which activates the automatic release of stress hormones. Next to the amygdala is the hippocampus, which creates memories.

- **The Cerebral Cortex Frontal Lobes:** Located behind our forehead and at the top of our head, the two sides of the cerebrum resemble a large walnut. This is the part of our brain that creates our conscious thinking. It plays a vital role in learning to manage the stress response.

The Spinal Cord

Our spinal cord can be thought of as an extension of the brain. Exiting through an opening at the base of our skull, the spinal cord is protected by the bones of the spinal column. Extending down the back, the spinal cord carries mental impulses from the brain to the body. Nerves exiting between the bones of the spinal column deliver operating instructions to every cell and organ of our body.

The Vagus Nerve

The vagus nerve can be thought of as a "second" spinal cord. But unlike the spinal cord, the vagus nerve isn't enclosed within the bones of the spinal column — it's free to roam throughout the body.

The word *vagus* comes from the Latin word meaning *wanderer,* which describes how the vagus nerve exits the brain and wanders down the front of the body. After leaving the skull, the vagus nerve divides into a right and left section. It delivers operating instructions that control the automatic functions of the body, such as breathing, heart rate, and kidney function.

The vagus nerve can do two different things:

- It can stimulate automatic functions that put us into fight-or-flight.

- It can relax automatic functions, which puts us into rest-and-digest.

Because the vagus nerve controls whether we are in fight-or-flight or rest and digest, improving vagal tone helps us achieve and maintain a relaxed state of being. The next chapter explains simple things we can do to tone our vagus nerve that will help us live our lives in a more relaxed state of being.

The Takeaway

Responses triggered by the vagus nerve are natural and fully automatic. The vagus nerve determines whether we are in fight-or-flight or rest and digest. Becoming aware and understanding what is happening will help us respond to challenges with more clarity and control.

Chapter Three

Improving Vagal Tone

Improving vagal tone can:

- Help you feel more relaxed

- Help you sleep better

- Reduce the risk of heart disease

- Improve digestive health

Singing and Sound-Based Techniques

The vagus nerve wanders down the back of our throat and connects to our vocal cords. We can stimulate the vagus nerve and increase vagal tone by singing.

Singing has been shown to lower stress, improve lung function, lift our mood, and help us cope with life's challenges. Singing and humming can stimulate the vagus nerve, enhance vagal tone, and strengthen the body's ability to respond to stress. Joining a chorus, singing in your car, or singing in the shower are all easy ways to incorporate singing into your life.

I remember suggesting to a patient suffering from stress to sing on the way home after getting an adjustment to help his body stay in a relaxed state of being.

"I can't sing!" he said.

I told him about "Johnny One Note." This story made him laugh, and hopefully, he sang a note or two on his way home that day.

Johnny One Note

"Johnny One Note" is the title of a song from the 1937 musical, *Babes in Arms,* written by Rodgers and Hammerstein and recorded by Judy Garland. The song is about a young opera singer named Johnny who could only sing one note, but he sang that one note with enthusiasm and power!

The Role of Laughter

If you can laugh at yourself,
you will never cease to be amused.

—The Dalai Lama, who also said he sometimes
considers himself "a professional laugher."

The largest concentration of vagus nerve branches is located in the abdomen, and a good belly laugh is an excellent way to improve vagal tone.

People who like to laugh can become certified laughing instructors who lead groups of people in voluntary laughter. Some of these instructors call what they do "Laughter Yoga." You can search YouTube for Laughter Yoga videos. Some are quite hilarious and you may find yourself laughing along. Laughter is a creative and unexpected way to lift your mood, as demonstrated by Laughter Yoga participants worldwide.

I remember seeing one group leader who had the participants pretend they were starting their lawn mower. With each pull of the cord, they all said "Ha!" and when the instructor's lawn mower started, all the lawn mowers started. The participants pushed their imaginary lawn mowers around the room, laughing all the way. Another exercise was having the participants open their credit card bills. As they looked at the imaginary statement they were holding in front of them, they all began laughing out loud.

Getting together with a group of people to laugh sounds like a funny thing to do, but that's the point. It may sound unconventional, but that's the beauty of it: laughter is healing. Sounds like a good party theme to me!

Norman Cousins

Norman Cousins, born in 1915, was an American journalist best known for his personal experiment of using humor for healing. When he was diagnosed with ankylosing spondylitis, an autoimmune disease leading to chronic inflammatory arthritis, doctors told him he had only a slim chance of recovery. Cousins began using laughter therapy — including watching funny movies, such as the Marx Brothers — to help his body heal.

In 1979, after recovering from his illness, Cousins wrote a book, titled *"Anatomy of an Illness,"* which helped raise awareness of how emotions and attitudes play a role in physical health. His views about health and healing helped shape scientific thinking into a more holistic view of health. His experience showed how the steps we take to manage stress are just as important as the medical interventions for managing chronic illness.

The Takeaway

Improving vagal tone helps your body shift more easily from tension to peace.

The more tools we have to manage stress, the more power we have to maintain and improve our health. The next chapter explains other ways to regulate our body's stress response.

Chapter Four
Calming the Body

Mastering others is strength;
mastering yourself is true power.

—Tao Te Ching

Although closely related, mindfulness and meditation are two separate practices for reducing emotional stress naturally, without the use of alcohol, drugs, or other harmful substances and behaviors.

Using alcohol and drugs to manage emotional stress can be thought of as sinking *below* the level of thinking. Using mindfulness and meditation to manage stress can be thought of as *rising above* the level of thinking.

Mindfulness and meditation may sound like something you could never do, or maybe you tried, but felt frustrated. These two practices are easy to learn and could be precisely what you need to calm your body and mind.

Meditation

Meditation involves learning simple techniques for slowing the stream of thoughts flowing through our mind. According to Dr. Fred Luskin of Stanford University, the average person thinks about 60,000 thoughts each day, with 90 percent of these thoughts being repetitive. However, research from Queen's University in Ontario suggests people only think 6,200 thoughts per day. Still, that is a lot of thinking! And much of it can be described as "stinkin thinkin!"

Credited to an ancient Chinese philosopher, Lao Tzu, who thought to have lived in the 6th century BCE, the following idea illustrates not only the importance of becoming aware of our thinking, but also the need to learn how to manage our thoughts.

Thoughts become emotions, emotions become words, words become actions, actions become habits, habits become character, and character becomes destiny.

Becoming mindful slows the flow of racing thoughts, helps us relax, and enhances our overall sense of well-being. The best thing about mindfulness is that it can be practiced while we are doing our activities of daily living.

Mindfulness

Mindfulness is nothing more than giving your full attention to what you are doing and how you are feeling in the present moment. By simply observing, but not judging, you can become mindful by focusing on:

- The thoughts you are thinking

- The way you are feeling

- The way you are breathing

- Your surroundings

Becoming mindful is a skill worth learning, but as in learning any new skill, it takes practice and patience.

> *Whether you think you can or think you can't,*
> *you're right.*
>
> —Henry Ford

Sometimes, when a patient tells me they are under a lot of stress, I ask if they meditate or practice mindfulness. Some responses I get include:

- "I can't meditate! My mind is too active!"

- "I've heard of mindfulness, but I can't do that!"

My response is to ask them if they know how to breathe.

"Of course, I do," they say, looking at me, wondering why I would ask such a question.

I explain that if you can just observe your breath coming in and leaving your body, you are practicing being mindful.

Breathing Practices

Breathing is one of the body's automatic processes — and we rarely stop to think about it — but bringing awareness to our breathing is a powerful first step toward managing emotional stress.

From the first breath we take when we are born until the last breath we take when we die, our breath is our connection to life. When we are carefree babies, we breathe deeply, allowing our abdomen to expand as our lungs fill with the oxygen we need to survive and thrive. This type of breathing is called diaphragmatic breathing, or "belly breathing."

When we are under stress, breathing becomes shallow. We breathe into our upper chest rather than our abdomen. Take a few moments to observe your breathing. Are you taking nice, slow, deep breaths, or is your breathing shallow?

What You Can Do

Remembering how to breathe the way we used to breathe when we were babies is easy. Here's how:

1. Get comfortable, either sitting or lying down.

2. Place your hands on your abdomen and feel it expand as you slowly inhale through your nose.

3. As your lungs fill with air your upper chest will begin to expand also.

4. Slowly exhale through nose or mouth.

5. Repeat.

That's all there is to it. After a few minutes of focusing on breathing the way you used to breathe when you didn't have a care in the world, mindful breathing will become the best tool you can use for managing emotional stress.

Taking the time to learn how to breathe this way helps us in many ways, because:

- Focusing on the breath as it enters and leaves the body gives us something to concentrate on besides our worries and concerns.

- Muscles need oxygen to relax.

- Waste products from cells (carbon dioxide) are released during exhalation.

- Our brain, which uses more oxygen than any other organ in the body, needs oxygen to function properly.

To further support the nervous system, we can employ strategies such as "Box Breathing."

Navy SEAL Box Breathing

Box breathing reduces stress, improves focus, lowers heart rate, and promotes mindfulness. It's a technique practiced by Navy SEALs, athletes, and others who aim to stay calm and focused during challenging moments.

In all the yoga classes I've attended and all the self-help books I've read, I've never liked anyone telling me how to breathe. You may feel the same way, but Box Breathing is one practice I really like.

Here's how it's done:

1. Inhale through your nose four seconds.

2. Hold your breath four seconds.

3. Exhale through your mouth four seconds.

4. Hold the air out four seconds.

5. Repeat.

Other breathing practices you may want to try include:

- Visualize inhaling peace and exhaling stress.

- For increasing energy, make the inhalation longer than the exhalation.

- For relaxing, make the exhalation longer than the inhalation.

- Visualize inhaling pink positive energy and exhaling gray negative energy.

Mindful breathing techniques can become a *Superpower* for you because they give you direct access to your nervous system. They provide a powerful way to anchor yourself in the present moment and quiet the emotional storm that may be brewing inside. Relief from stress doesn't always require drastic measures. Sometimes a few mindful breaths are all it takes to turn chaos into calmness.

In the next chapter we will explore how mindfulness can be seamlessly integrated into everyday routines.

Chapter Five

Daily Mindfulness Techniques

As the following story demonstrates, mindfulness can be practiced anywhere, anytime, no matter what you are doing.

A generous person wanted to donate a dishwasher to a monastery so the monks wouldn't have to spend time washing dishes by hand. The monks appreciated the offer, but said, "No thank you." For them, washing dishes was a good way to practice mindfulness.

Focusing on washing dishes while consciously breathing and relaxing is a great example of practicing mindfulness during daily activities. Whether it's cleaning your home, building a piece of furniture, preparing a meal, gardening, or working in the yard, focusing on an activity you enjoy can be considered a mindful activity.

Other ways to practice mindfulness include:

Mindful Hydration

Instead of mindlessly pouring and gulping down a glass of water, sipping slowly, or savoring a cup of tea, is an easy way to practice mindfulness.

An example of drinking tea to achieve a peaceful state of being is the Japanese Tea Ceremony. This ceremony was developed as a *transformative practice* to help people relax and focus on inner peace. During the ceremony, the tea is prepared slowly and mindfully. From washing the teapot to waiting for the water to boil, each step is done with patience to fully immerse oneself in the present moment.

Eating

Slowing down to chew each bite – while noticing the color, texture, odor, and flavor of what you are eating — is an excellent mindfulness exercise.

Avoiding distractions such as looking at your phone, television, or working while eating, can improve digestion and help create healthier eating habits. Mindfulness when eating can include asking yourself some questions. What triggered you to eat? How did you feel after eating? Could you have made better choices?

Silent Walking

Silent walking as a way to practice mindfulness is nothing new. Many cultures, including Zen Buddhists, use walking meditations to quiet their minds and connect to the inner peace within. Some monks suggest we consider every step as an act of *kissing the earth* as a helpful way of becoming mindful.

Many years ago, I joined a small group that met at six every morning in a friend's living room. We would sit silently in a circle on the floor before starting our day. When the leader rang a soft bell, we silently stood, then walked outside in single file. We circled the pool a couple of times, returned inside, and sat back down again — without ever saying a word to each other. At the time, it felt a little odd, since not a single word was spoken the entire time we were there.

Looking back, I am grateful for the experience of learning about mindful walking, a practice that can be done anywhere, even inside your home or an office building whenever you need to quiet your mind.

The Healing Power of Nature

Spending time in nature improves our sense of well-being. A visit to the beach, mountains, forest, park, or even the backyard, can quiet our minds and reduce stress and anxiety. Spending time in nature can also give rise to creative ideas and insights. Taking time to admire a beautiful sunset, or stars in the sky at night are mindful activities.

Taking a break from the constant input of electronic devices and allowing our senses to fully engage in the environment is an opportunity for introspection and self-reflection, important activities that are often neglected.

The Butterfly Hug

A mindful technique taught by mental-health professionals to regulate the stress response is called the butterfly hug. It is performed by crossing the arms over the chest and placing the hands at the level of the collar bones.

Next, begin gently tapping the hands one at a time, — left, right, left, right — creating a slow rhythm from side to side. The butterfly hug can be done anytime we feel stressed.

Aromatherapy

Our nose has olfactory bulbs that are connected to our limbic system, the part of our brain that controls emotions, memories, and mood. Aromatherapy is the practice of inhaling the scent of essential oils derived from plants to help manage emotional stress. Inhaling scents such as lavender and chamomile have been shown to lower cortisol levels, activate our rest and digest mode, reduce heart rate, and improve sleep.

Using a diffuser to add scent to your space or putting a little lavender oil on your bed pillow can be a mindful bedtime ritual that soothes and helps you unwind.

A 2016 review in the *Journal of Advanced Nursing* found that inhaling the scent of lavender essential oil reduced anxiety in patients undergoing various medical procedures. Other studies suggest that lavender oil improves the quality of sleep for people suffering from sleep disorders. Since the evidence is still being debated, more studies are needed.

Learning a new skill takes practice and effort, and the small improvements we feel will inspire us to keep moving forward in the journey of achieving more inner peace. Over time, practicing one, two, or more of the mindfulness techniques that appeal to you helps you build a powerful foundation of calm and clarity.

In the next chapter, we will explore the mystery of the human brain. Understanding the relationship between the conscious mind and the subconscious mind opens the door to mastering our mind rather than becoming the slave to automatic thoughts that cause tension and stress.

Chapter Six

The Human Mind is a Mystery

As a man thinketh, so he is.

Proverb 23:70

Closely linked to the brain, the mind includes things beyond the physical form such as beliefs, desires, and emotions. The workings of the human mind are a mystery that has been debated for centuries by psychologists, philosophers, neuroscientists, and mystics – but the question persists: Is the mind a byproduct of brain activity, or is it something more? As experts debate the complexities of the human mind, they all agree our mind operates as if it is divided into two main sections:

- The conscious mind

- The subconscious mind

The Conscious Mind

The conscious mind is our thinking mind, and it governs voluntary actions such as walking and speaking. Most conscious-mind activity takes place in the prefrontal cortex, the front part of our brain just behind our forehead. This part of our brain is the newest part of our brain to develop.

The conscious mind:

- Thinks things over

- Makes decisions

- Holds short-term memories

The Subconscious Mind

Like a computer program, the subconscious mind is always running in the background. It gathers data and provides a database that becomes the foundation for our thinking. From the moment of our birth (or maybe even before), every belief, habit, and emotion we have experienced, whether or not we remember it, is stored in our subconscious mind.

The subconscious mind:

- Records everything we've ever experienced

- Controls automatic processes of the body

- Gives rise to creative ideas and sudden realizations

Old beliefs, forgotten trauma, and unconscious fears are stored in our subconscious mind and give rise to patterns of negative self-talk. When we understand this, we can take steps to reprogram the subconscious mind by installing new, empowering mental programs.

Life experiences can lead us to believe we are not good enough or that we don't deserve to do well in life. These beliefs form the foundation of our thinking. They can influence the decisions we make and how we respond to the challenges of life.

The Takeaway

We can learn to use our conscious mind to reprogram our subconscious mind. We can replace negative beliefs that prevent us from becoming the best version of ourselves we can be.

The following chapter explains how we can reprogram our subconscious mind. We can become the master of our mind rather than being a slave to limiting beliefs. It takes some time and effort, but it can be done.

Chapter Seven
Reprogramming Thought Patterns

The mind is a garden, and thoughts are the seeds. You can grow flowers, or you can grow weeds.

Some say the *spelling of words* refers to how our words cast a spell over our lives. That may or may not be true, but the words we speak have power.

When patients come into my office and say things such as:

- "I can't relax."

- "I'm falling apart."

- "I'm a mess."

I stop them in their tracks, look them in the eyes, and use my fake stern voice to say, "Please!"

After getting their full attention, I add, "Please do not talk like that in my office! Why don't you say something positive, such as how grateful you are that you have a good chiropractor?"

This often gets a chuckle, as people realize their words are not helping them, but could be hurting them.

Affirmations

Affirmations are positive statements we can repeat to ourselves that, over time, help replace negative programming in our subconscious mind. You can say them out loud or say them to yourself in your head. The key to using affirmations is to:

- Believe what you are saying is true.

- Feel what you are saying is true.

- Know what you are saying is true.

Affirmations can encourage, motivate, and help us overcome negative thinking. They work by installing "new files" that build self-confidence, reinforce positive habits, and improve our overall attitude. Quieting the conscious mind allows greater access to the subconscious, making it easier to install new beliefs and patterns of thinking.

Neuroplasticity

Neuroplasticity describes the brain's ability to change and adapt by forming new connections between neurons.

For decades, psychologists and scientists thought the human brain of an adult was hardwired, set in its ways, and unable to change. But that isn't true. Our thought processes are not fixed. They can be changed. We can rewire our brain and change how we think.

Challenge yourself

The greatest weapon against stress is our ability to choose one thought over another.

—William James

If we are accustomed to thinking negative thoughts, we can start by challenging ourselves. If you catch yourself saying or thinking a negative statement about yourself, ask yourself:

- Is this something I would say to a friend?

- Is this 100 percent true?

- Is there a more helpful way of looking at this?

For people who are accustomed to negative self-talk, I suggest gentle affirmations such as:

- "I am beginning to understand the power my words have over my health."

- "I am open to changing the way I think and speak."

What You Can Do

There are many ways to use affirmations effectively, including:

- Repeat them every day, either out loud or in your mind.

- Say them with confidence and emotion.

- Place them where you can see them.

- Say them to yourself while looking at yourself in a mirror.

- Record them on your phone and listen while relaxing.

- Listen to affirmations recorded by others.

You can use or modify some of the affirmations listed below or create your own. Adding gratitude makes affirmations even more powerful. An example would be, "I am grateful for my inner peace and sense of well-being."

Affirmations for Managing Stress

- With each breath, I am becoming calm and relaxed.

- I am letting go of things I cannot control.

- Everything is in divine order.

- I deserve peace, joy, and balance.

- I respond to challenges with calmness.

- I am strong and resilient.

- I am doing my best and that is enough.

I am Safe

One of the most powerful affirmations we can say is, "I am safe." Making this simple statement — while believing it and feeling it — changes our state of being from fight-or-flight to rest and digest.

We've all experienced traumatic events in our lives. Thoughts and feelings associated with these events have been recorded by our subconscious mind. If we are safe in the present moment, reminding ourselves that we are safe allows our body and mind to relax.

Visualization

Visualization is a technique where you close your eyes and use your imagination to create a picture in your mind that relaxes you. You could visualize yourself standing on the shore of a beautiful ocean, walking on a trail in a forest, standing on a mountain top, or sitting by a fireplace in a cozy cabin in the woods. Our imagination is a powerful tool we can use to help move from fight-or-flight to a more relaxed state of being.

Our subconscious mind cannot tell the difference between what is happening in our lives and what is happening in our "magic nation." As you imagine your favorite scene, your body will begin to relax. For example, using all your senses, picture yourself standing on a warm, sun-drenched shoreline. Imagine the rhythm of the gentle waves sliding onto the shore, calming your body. Feel your worries being taken away by the whispering ocean breeze. Imagine breathing in the scent of salt water air and feel the sand under your feet.

Other visualization techniques include:

- Visualize your troublesome thoughts as clouds passing by.

- Visualize your worries as leaves, falling into a river and being carried away.

- Imagine standing under a waterfall. As the water gently falls upon you, your stress is washed away into the flowing river.

- Before making a presentation or some other stressful event, imagine yourself doing a great job.

Affirmations are a gentle yet powerful way to rewire your subconscious mind. They can help align your mind with the life you want to create. When our conscious mind is quiet and our body is relaxed, the subconscious mind is open to receiving suggestions and creating new thought patterns.

The next chapter will explain how hypnosis is nothing more than a relaxed and focused state of being.

Chapter Eight

Hypnosis

The word hypnosis was coined in 1842 by James Braid, a surgeon who lulled his patients into a deep state of relaxation. His treatment included filling the minds of his patients with healing suggestions and affirmations.

Hypnosis comes from the Greek word *hypnos,* which means 'sleep,' although those who are lulled into a state of hypnosis are not actually sleeping. They are just deeply relaxed. Feeling as if their body is sleeping, their conscious mind is quiet, but their subconscious mind is alert and focused.

When Braid realized his patients were not really sleeping, it was too late. The word *hypnosis* was already being used by others practicing the same art, and the term stuck.

Hollywood has given hypnosis a bad reputation. The idea of being hypnotized gives many people the creeps. However, for some, the chance to get on stage, shed their inhibitions, and bark like a dog or speak like a Martian sounds like fun. When a stage hypnotist asks a volunteer to come up on stage, they willingly do what the hypnotist asks them to do. However, a hypnotist cannot make a person do anything that goes against their moral code.

Hypnosis Helped Mayo Clinic

In the early 1900s, the death rate from new chemical anesthetics such as ether and chloroform was high. Many patients died during surgical procedures at other hospitals during those early years. But thanks to a nurse anesthesiologist by the name of Alice Magaw, the Mayo brothers had more successful outcomes.

Nurse Magaw used hypnosis to help patients achieve a deep state of relaxation before and during surgery, and less anesthesia was needed. The willingness to try new and unconventional methods with patients played a significant but often overlooked role in making the Mayo Clinic famous.

Slowing Down Brain Waves

Brain waves are electrical impulses produced by the activity of brain cells. They have different frequencies and are categorized by the speed of their impulses. There are several types of brain waves:

- Delta waves are the slowest waveforms. They are associated with deep sleep.

- Theta waves are associated with deep relaxation, light sleep, and creativity.

- Alpha waves are associated with relaxed but alert states, such as meditation and day dreaming.

- Beta waves occur when we are thinking and solving problems.

- Gamma Waves are the fastest waves. They are associated with peak mental and spiritual states.

Breathing techniques and mindfulness can slow down our brainwaves and help us achieve deep states of relaxation. It is during these moments of quiet relaxation that the subconscious mind can easily accept new thought patterns.

Some people hire a hypnotherapist to help them achieve goals such as losing weight or quitting smoking. During a hypnotherapy session, the therapist guides the client into a deep state of relaxation. When the body is relaxed and brain waves slow down, the subconscious mind becomes receptive to receiving suggestions and affirmations.

Quiet moments of relaxation are the perfect time for listening to recorded affirmations, speaking them aloud, or saying them to yourself in your mind. The following self-relaxation technique can be used to relax the body and mind and make affirmations more effective.

Autogenic Training

Autogenic training is a method of using the mind to reduce tension and stress. Developed in the 1920s by German psychologist Johannes Schultz, it can be used to relax the body and mind. The steps are easy to follow and can be modified to your preferences.

1. Lie down and make yourself comfortable. Place a pillow under your knees to take pressure off the low back. If desired, also place a small pillow under your neck.

2. Begin by breathing in through your nose and exhaling through your mouth or nose. As you inhale, feel your abdomen rise and your chest expand. This ensures the breath is full and complete rather than shallow.

3. Begin using your mind to relax your body by saying to yourself, "My left arm is heavy." You can repeat this phrase several times as you feel your arm becoming heavy.

4. Next, say to yourself, "My right arm is heavy." Repeat a few times.

5. Proceed through every section of your body, breathing slowly and deeply and making your body feel heavy. Very, very heavy….

6. Next, repeat the process with the left arm and make each body part feel warm. "My left arm is warm. My right arm is warm." By the time you reach your feet and toes, your entire body will feel heavy, warm, and quite relaxed.

7. If your mind drifts off to other things during the process, simply take note of the thought and return your thoughts to your breathing. Become totally aware of your breathing. Observe your breath as it enters and leaves through your nose.

8. If something from the past comes to mind, use your breathing to inhale the future and release the past. Feel yourself totally in the present moment, breathing and relaxing.

It is possible to achieve a deep state of relaxation while doing this. To end the session, it is a good idea to wiggle your toes, open and close your hands, and then open your eyes to end the session.

Highway Hypnosis

Highway hypnosis occurs when someone driving a car seems unaware of what they are doing. It is a mental state during which the conscious mind quiets down and the subconscious mind is alert.

Highway hypnosis can happen when the driver is over-tired, mentally overloaded, or if there is a lack of sensory stimulation to keep the conscious mind alert. The driver enters a trance-like state where conscious thoughts quiet down. Detaching from the immediate surroundings, the subconscious remains active and takes over the task of driving. This can be dangerous. It can lead to falling asleep at the wheel, slower reaction times, or missing an exit. But it demonstrates how powerful and efficient the subconscious mind can be.

The Takeaway

Hypnosis is an altered state of being during which the conscious mind is quiet and the subconscious mind is alert. During this state of being, the brain can be rewired with new patterns of thinking.

In the next chapter, heart-brain coherence, another easy-to-learn powerful state of being for relaxing the body and mind will be discussed.

Chapter Nine

The HeartMath Institute

The HeartMath Institute is a non-profit organization that develops methods to help people achieve well-being by regulating the flow of nerve impulses between the heart and the brain.

As the command center of the body, the brain sends signals to the heart, but the heart has its own electrical system and also sends signals to the brain. In fact, the heart sends more signals to the brain than the brain sends to the heart.

Balancing this flow of energy is known as heart-brain coherence. When the circulation of neural impulses between the brain and the heart is balanced, the harmonious state of being can:

- Reduce emotional stress

- Lower blood pressure

- Improve our quality of sleep

- Improve creative thinking

When the circulation of energy between the brain and the heart is out of tune, it can trigger emotions associated with the stress response, including:

- Fear

- Anger

- Anxiety

- Worry

- Stress-related health problems

A HeartMath Exercise

The HeartMath Institute teaches a simple exercise to achieve heart-brain coherence. Performing the exercise creates a smooth wave-like energy pattern indicating balance between the heart and brain. Heart-brain coherence creates feelings of love, compassion, and gratitude.

The following exercise quiets the thinking mind, opens the heart, and creates heart-brain coherence. The steps are as follows:

- Put your hand or hands over your heart.

- Imagine breathing into your heart.

- Think of someone or something you love or something for which you are grateful.

When I suggest this technique to patients, I don't ask them to tell me what they love, but sometimes they do. Two recent declarations of love made me smile.

"I love my bed!" said one with a big smile on her face.

Another patient said, "I love goats in pajamas!"

I wasn't sure what she meant by that, and I didn't ask for details. After she left my office, I had a free moment, so I Googled it and discovered videos of baby goats, dressed in pajamas romping around. It's as if they are having a pajama party. I loved it too!

Promoting Global Coherence

In collaboration with Dr. Joe Dispenza, known for his work on the mind-body connection, the HeartMath Institute conducts research to measure electrical energy emitted by the body. According to their research, published in peer-reviewed scientific journals, the body's energy field can be measured and has been found to extend several feet outside the body.

The scientific community has debated claims about energy fields extending beyond the body, but combining biophysics and quantum biology is an emerging field of scientific study. The National Institute of Health refers to this as subtle energy fields or biofield therapies.

Based on their research findings, the HeartMath Institute believes teaching people to achieve heart-brain coherence can result in a positive chain reaction. People who practice heart-brain coherence can emit energy to help others feel peace and harmony. This can lead to improved global harmony for dealing with challenges facing humanity.

Suppose future technology allows scientists to measure subtle energy fields. In that case, the goals of the HeartMath Institute for spreading peace and love across the globe will be recognized and celebrated, and a quote often attributed to Mahatma Gandhi could apply:

First, they ignore you, then they laugh at you, then they fight you, then you win.

The Takeaway

Heart-brain coherence is a powerful state of being for reducing stress and achieving emotional balance. Synchronizing the heart and brain through techniques such as heart-focused breathing, helps move the body into a state of harmony. By tapping into this inner alignment, we can learn to respond to the challenges of life with greater calm and clarity, one heartbeat and one breath at a time.

Rather than focusing on the thoughts in our heads, we can learn to achieve heart-brain coherence. As more people do the same, more heart-to-heart conversations can create an atmosphere of compassion and understanding.

Chapter Ten

Emotional Triggers

Emotional triggers are automatic responses to something we see, hear, or think. They create strong reactions such as fear, anger, sadness, or insecurity. These emotions, which could be caused by emotions stored in the subconscious mind, need to be processed and released.

Learning how to regulate the automatic response to an emotional trigger is possible. The first step is becoming aware of feelings and emotions that arise when triggered.

Scan, Sense, Soothe

Have you ever noticed how your body reacts to an emotional trigger even before your mind catches up? Becoming aware of the physical sensations that arise when we are triggered helps us step back and observe the situation. This gives us the opportunity to use our conscious mind to decide how to act, rather than automatically reacting.

When you are triggered, take a few moments to perform the following body scan:

- Direct your attention to different parts of your body, such as your neck, chest, or back.

- Notice any tension, numbness or other sensations.

- Describe how it feels. Is it tight? Warm?

- Respond with compassion to these feelings by directing your breathing to that area, or gently moving or stretching that part of your body.

Name it to Tame it

Dr. Dan Siegel, a professor of psychiatry at the UCLA School of Medicine, coined the phrase – "Name it to tame it." It is based on becoming aware and recognizing our emotions. By doing so, we can use our rational thinking brain to regulate our responses.

The key to handling emotional triggers is learning not to overreact. When you feel triggered, try using the pause technique. Here's how:

- When you feel emotions being activated, realize you are being triggered.

- Take a moment or two and think of the word *Pause*.

- Take a few deep breaths.

- Ask yourself if your reaction is from now, or from the past.

- Instead of being impulsive and over-reacting, respond calmly.

We can learn to recognize when emotional triggers bring unresolved emotions to the surface. This helps us act with clarity and choice rather than reacting. By learning to pause, think, and choose our response, we reclaim our power and give space to our healing and growth.

Chapter Eleven
Processing Emotions

Between stimulus and response, there is a space.
In that space is our power to choose our response.
In our response lies our growth and freedom.

—Victor Frankl, Holocaust survivor and author of
"Man's Search for Meaning."

In his poem "The Guest House," Rumi, a 13th-century poet, says that a human being is a guest house and emotions are visitors. Some are joyful, some are mean, and some arrive in groups, filling our home with sorrow.

We never know what emotions might show up at our front door. Rumi says we should meet them at the door, welcome them with a smile, and invite them into our home. We should treat them with honor because they may have been sent as a guide from beyond. They may be clearing us out for some new delight.

Many people turn to alcohol, drugs, and other harmful behaviors to suppress negative emotions when they arise. Rather than suppressing them, we can view these visitors as emotions that want to be recognized. Thinking of these emotions this way allows us to relax, breathe, and give them the space and time they need to dissipate.

Processing negative emotions as they arise requires awareness, self-compassion, and practical tools. There are many ways to process and release negative emotions when they arise. Different techniques work better for some than others. For some people, crying, talking, or writing about these feelings helps process them.

Crying

Weeping may linger for the night,
but joy comes with the morning.

Psalm 30:5

We usually associate crying with feeling sad, but according to an article in *Harvard Health,* crying helps us release emotional stress.

Crying in response to irritants to the eyes contain mostly water, but tears shed in response to emotional stress contain some stress hormones. Crying acts like a safety valve. It releases stress hormones and activates the parasympathetic nervous system. This causes the release of happy hormones such as oxytocin and endorphins to help us feel better.

In the 1987 movie *Broadcast News*, Holly Hunter played a woman who had a high-stress job in television news. Although she is successful and brilliant at her job, she spends a few moments each day crying. This is her way of releasing stress. This demonstrates how crying can be used to process stressful emotions.

If you feel better after crying, it can be a helpful coping mechanism. Everyone is different. Some people feel worse after crying. If crying happens too often or becomes uncontrollable, a mental-health professional should be consulted for evaluation and treatment.

Venting

For some people, talking to a friend can be a powerful tool for processing emotions. Sometimes, just knowing someone cares enough to listen to you can bring a huge relief.

Ideally, as you share what you're feeling and thinking, the person you are venting to will offer comfort, understanding, or maybe a new perspective. Having a trusted friend who will listen is a gift to be treasured, and returning the favor when your friend needs to vent can deepen the trust between you.

Some people think talking about your emotions when you are stressed gives those emotions more power and should not be discussed with anyone. But if you need to talk, then you need to talk. If you do not feel comfortable talking about your emotions with someone you know, talking to a mental-health counselor — as will be discussed at the end of this chapter — can be helpful. An alternative

to talking about your feelings is to vent by writing in a
journal.

Journaling

Writing things down can be a powerful tool for reducing
emotional stress. Writing about how we feel creates space
between us and our emotions. Taking a few minutes to jot
down your thoughts can reduce overwhelm and provide
clarity.

Spending a few minutes writing down what you feel —
without censoring yourself or worrying about spelling or
grammar — can be helpful. When finished, you can either
keep the journal or tear it up. Either way is okay.

Cold Water

Using cold water to process and reduce emotional stress
has been used for centuries. From the ancient Romans and
Greeks who incorporated ice plunges into their bath house
rituals, to the Japanese purification ritual of standing
under a cold waterfall, using cold water to reduce emotional stress has deep roots in many cultures.

Cold water activates the parasympathetic nervous
system. This helps move us from fight-or-flight to
rest-and-digest. Some people use cold baths and showers
as a regular part of their self-care. Reasons range from
elevating mood, boosting energy, building resilience, and
bringing us fully into the present moment.

Everyone is different, and for many people, taking a cold shower to reduce stress is not very appealing. For some, taking a warm shower relaxes them.

Shake It Off

To burn off stress hormones and return to a more relaxed state of being, some animals naturally shake it off. In a video available online, a polar bear is seen running away from a helicopter following it from the sky. When the helicopter gets close enough, researchers fire a dart from a rifle causing the polar bear to fall into the snow and lose consciousness.

After the researchers finish their examination of the bear, they stand by and watch as the polar bear returns to a waking state. As the bear wakes up, he begins shaking his entire body as if having a seizure. As the researchers explain, the bear's shaking is a way to burn off adrenaline and stress hormones produced during the stress response.

If our stress response has been activated when there is no threat of physical danger, we can turn on some music and shake it off. Dancing to music or shaking our body regulates the stress response by burning off the adrenaline and cortisol.

As will be discussed in a later chapter, this story of the polar bear illustrates the work of Dr. Peter Levine, who developed a mental-health technique called Somatic Experiencing (SE).

Emotional Freedom Technique (EFT)

Emotional Freedom Technique (EFT) involves using your finger tips to gently tap on specific acupressure points on the face and upper body while focusing on a stressful emotion or symptom — and then going through the process again while focusing on the feeling of relief.

Combining acupressure on acupuncture points with cognitive reframing, tapping reduces physical stress and helps process the emotion rather than suppressing it.

Founded and developed by Gary Craig, a Stanford-educated engineer, EFT is an easy to learn self-care method based on the work of American psychologist Dr. Roger Callahan who knew about acupuncture points and used it to help a woman suffering from a water phobia in the 1980's.

Acupuncture, which dates back 2500 years ago, is based on the belief that life force flows through the body via pathways, called meridians, and that an imbalance of this flow causes emotional and physical stress.

Although many research and clinical studies show benefits of EFT for people suffering with stress and over-whelm, worry and anxiety, PTSD, pain, and phobias, scientists are skeptical due to lack of scientific proof that acupuncture meridians exist.

Millions of people like and use EFT because it's easy to learn, simple to use, can be done anywhere, and works quickly for balancing emotions.

For serious anxiety, trauma, or pain, it is best used as a complementary treatment alongside professional care – not to replace it.

There are many YouTube channels and videos explaining how to incorporate tapping into your self-care routine including:

- Nick Ortner – author of The Tapping Solution

- TapWithBrad

- Dr. Peta Stapleton, a psychologist in Australia who gave a presentation on EFT for Tedx and is involved in clinical research of the method.

Let It Go

*Sometimes, it takes a lot of effort to realize
life was meant to be effortless.*

I once had a patient who illustrates the power of letting go of stressful emotions. She worked a stressful job and would come to see me for an adjustment once a week. Although she would feel better for a day or two after her visit, she was not holding her adjustments and needed to come back every week. I suggested things she could do to reduce her stress, such as counseling, yoga, deep-breathing exercises, reducing caffeine, and even taking a warm bath at night to help release the tension in her muscles.

Nothing I suggested appealed to her. The best she could do was get a chiropractic adjustment for some temporary relief. One day, she arrived for her appointment and I could see a difference. She seemed relaxed. In fact, she seemed quite relaxed and was anxious to tell me what happened to her. She told me she went to her church, talked to the pastor, and then attended the service on Easter Sunday.

"I looked at Jesus on the cross and turned all my problems over to him," she said.

And obviously, she had done just that. I was amazed at the drastic change from one week to the next. She only needed a few minor adjustments that day. She made her usual appointment for the next week. When she came back a week later, she had maintained her sense of serenity and was holding her adjustments. She said she decided to quit her job and go to work for her church. She found a way to let it go.

The Takeaway

It is better to process emotions rather than suppress them. Suppressing emotions can cause physical pain. Facing our emotions with courage and honesty, giving them space, and allowing them to be released leads to healing.

Chapter Twelve

Resilience and Reframing

*It's not what happens to you
but how you react to it that matters.*

—Epictetus

Resilience is the ability to adapt and move forward when faced with challenges in life. It helps us heal and adapt to loss and failure. Being resilient helps us accept what happens without becoming overwhelmed or giving up.

An important tool in cultivating resilience is reframing. This involves changing the way we think about a situation by looking at it from a more helpful perspective. It doesn't mean denying that the situation is difficult; it just means shifting our mindset to change how we perceive a situation or an event. We can use our thinking mind to *zoom out* and find a way to see the experience in a more positive or helpful way.

Who's to Say What's Good or Bad?

There is an old story about a poor farmer that illustrates the power of reframing what events mean for us. The story begins with the farmer's horse running away. His neighbor thought that was terrible, but the farmer said, "Maybe yes, maybe no — who's to say?"

When his horse returned the next day bringing three wild horses with it, his neighbor thought it was wonderful. But again, the farmer said, "Maybe yes, maybe no — who's to say?"

When his son broke his leg trying to tame one of the wild horses, his neighbor thought it was terrible. Again, the farmer said, "Maybe yes, maybe no — who's to say?"

The next week, soldiers came by to draft young men to fight a war, but the farmer's son couldn't go because of his broken leg. The neighbor thought it was fortunate, but the farmer had the same response, "Maybe yes, maybe no — who's to say?"

Accepting the changes that happen to us during our lives and changing our perceptions by reframing them can be helpful. Sometimes, we need to zoom out and look at the bigger picture, rather than focusing solely on the event that happened. For example:

Instead of saying "I'm a failure" after losing a job, look at the situation as an opportunity to explore new opportunities or a new career.

Instead of stressing out while stuck in traffic, take a mindful breath and reframe it as having extra time to relax and breathe or listen to a podcast.

Instead of saying, "I really messed up" after making a mistake, reframe it as an opportunity to learn what to do or not do next time.

Instead of saying, "I'm worried. I don't know what's going to happen in the future," try reframing by looking at change as an opportunity for growth and new experiences.

Instead of saying, "He or she is so awful. I can't stand being around them," try reframing it by realizing they may be going through a difficult time in their life, or they may be limited in their ability to relate.

Instead of saying, "Today was horrible," try reframing it by telling yourself that you did the best you could do and tomorrow is a new day.

Instead of complaining about the way things are, take a moment to be grateful for the blessings you have.

Living the Dream

Want what you have, love what you do,
enjoy being who you are.

Recently, a patient came to my office, and when I asked him how he was doing, he replied that he was living the dream. I waited for what he was going to say next, thinking maybe he had won the lottery, got a new job or something spectacular had happened.

"What happened?" I asked.

"Living the dream," he repeated, smiling. "I have a roof over my head, a bed to sleep in, food in my pantry and clothes to wear. That's a lot better than a lot of people in the world today."

Gratitude

Gratitude is the magic formula you have been seeking.
—Abraham Hicks

According to scientific research in psychology and medicine, gratitude has been shown to reduce cortisol levels. Gratitude reduces stress and anxiety, and helps us sleep better. It also boosts our immune system. Taking a few minutes each day to count our blessings can go a long way in improving our lives, our relationships, and our health.

Keeping a gratitude journal and writing down two or three things we are grateful for each day helps us focus on the positive aspects of our life. By highlighting what is working well, gratitude can help us manage the challenges of life.

Chapter Thirteen

When to Seek Help

Sometimes, even though we may have a roof over our head, a bed to sleep in, food in our pantry, clothes to wear, and people to live with, the ups and downs of life may leave us feeling emotionally exhausted.

Life situations such as caregiving, being in an abusive relationship, workplace burnout, or an inability to deal with the pressures of life on earth can make it seem impossible to manage emotional stress.

Taking a mental-health day can sometimes help, but if feelings of helplessness, fear, guilt, resentment, failure, sadness, jealousy, anger, or other emotions persist or overwhelm, professional mental-health therapy can help. There are many new mental-health techniques available. Some have been shown to be effective with just a few visits, and many are available for online or telephone appointments.

The Top-Down Approach

Changing the thoughts in our heads to regulate our stress response and improve our emotional health has been the cornerstone of mental-health therapy for decades. This top-down approach to helping clients is often called talk therapy. It helps people improve their ability to manage stress. An example of talk therapy used by mental-health therapists includes:

- **Cognitive Behavioral Therapy (CBT)** is a form of talk therapy that helps people change their negative or inaccurate thought patterns about life situations that cause stress. CBT helps with conditions including depression, anxiety, and post-traumatic stress disorder. It is the most widely practiced mental health treatment.

- **Person-centered Therapy** is an approach that prioritizes the client's needs in a supportive and non-judgmental setting, without providing direction. Instead, the client is empowered to find their own solutions which builds self-awareness and confidence. Creating a strong trusting partnership between client and therapist is essential in this approach.

Other Brain-Based Techniques

The field of psychology has evolved to include other brain-based techniques. These forms of mental health therapy techniques are the fastest growing area in psychology. They have been shown to help release stored emotional trauma that sometimes takes years of talk therapy to heal.

Brain-based techniques focus on changing our physical state of being as a way of regulating the stress response in our brain.

The Polyvagal Theory

This brain-based way of dealing with mental-health issues was introduced to the Society of Psychophysiological Research in 1994 by Dr. Stephen Porges, an American neuropsychologist. His discovery redefined the relationship between the vagus nerve and stress.

The vagus nerve provides a highway for communication between the mind and body. It plays a role in determining our state of being. Rather than just fight-or-flight or rest-and-digest, Porges identified a third state of being. This newly discovered state of being is known as ventral vagal or safe and social.

Believed to be a newer branch of the vagus nerve, the ventral vagal state helps us feel safe, connected, and calm. It is the healthiest state of being. It supports our ability to regulate our emotions and our ability to get along with others.

Porges said there are three ways of being in the world:

- In the first stage, we are relaxed and can relate and communicate with others in a healthy way.

- In the second state, our fight-or-flight response is activated.

- In the third state, which Porges calls *shutdown*, overwhelming stress causes a person to detach and withdraw. If provoked, they can unleash bursts of anger, or worse.

The Polyvagal Theory explains how emotional and physical stress affects the vagus nerve and how practices such as breathing and singing can restore vagal tone. Some brain-based techniques are being used today to treat post-traumatic stress disorder (PTSD) and other stress-related emotional issues.

EMDR

Eye Movement Desensitization and Reprocessing Therapy (EMDR) is an evidence-based therapy developed by Dr. Francine Shapiro in 1987. It is used to treat PTSD and phobias. EMDR has been associated with reducing the impact of the memory associated with the traumatic event.

Administered by a mental-health care professional, the patient is encouraged to bring a traumatic event to mind that needs to be released. The process involves bilateral stimulation which can be achieved by following the finger of the therapist moving back and forth. Wearing headphones with a soft beeping sound alternating from one ear to the other can also be used.

Brainspotting

Developed by Dr. David Grand, a licensed clinical social worker with a Ph.D. from the International University, Brainspotting combines body awareness and eye position to process trauma.

The method involves helping the patient find an eye position, while physical and emotional sensations are observed. Not a lot of talking is required. The therapist simply supports the process of finding where the tension is held. The technique involves helping the client release trauma, anxiety and other emotional blocks to optimal functioning.

Somatic Experiencing

Developed by Dr. Peter Levine, an American psychotherapist, Somatic Experiencing (SE) is an approach to healing stress and trauma that has brought attention to body-mind medicine. With doctorates in both medical biophysics and psychology, Dr. Levine was able to understand how trauma and stress affect the nervous system.

SE involves becoming aware of how you feel physically. Through various techniques such as stretching, breathing, and shaking, energy stored in the body from traumatic events is located and released. SE is used to treat PTSD, chronic pain, and other stress-related disorders.

How to Find a Therapist

There are many options for finding a therapist to work with you. You can ask your primary-care doctor, check with your insurance carrier or go to PsychologyToday.com and use the filters to find therapists in your area.

If a therapist is familiar with several different techniques, they will be able to develop a treatment plan that will work best for you. In addition to therapy, medications are sometimes needed to manage emotional stress.

Many health professionals have YouTube channels where they discuss and sometimes demonstrate their techniques, which could be a good starting point for learning about available options. There are also online directories for finding a specific type of therapist, such as

Somatic therapy directory:
https://directory.traumahealing.org

EMDR International Association:
https://www.emdria.org/find-an-emdr-therapist

Brain Spotting Directory
https://brainspotting.com/directory

Working on our mental health is just as important as working on our physical health, financial health, and every other area of our lives.

Professional therapy is a valuable tool that can increase self-awareness, provide helpful guidance for navigating life's challenges, and open the door to healing and growth.

Part II

Chemical Stress

Chemical stress comes from the foods we eat, the products we use, and the environment around us. These toxins disrupt our hormones, drain our energy, and weaken our immune system.

This section shares simple, practical ways to reduce chemical stress in daily life.

Chemical stress feeds physical stress by triggering inflammation that leads to pain and discomfort – and when the body is strained, emotional stress soon follows.

The good news is, you can break the cycle.

Small consistent changes such as choosing cleaner food and pure water can make a big difference. Better food and water can help your body restore balance and awaken your body's natural healing power.

Chapter Fourteen

Chemicals in Our Food

Today in the United States, there are more than 10,000 chemicals approved by the Food and Drug Administration (FDA) to be used in food, food processing, and food packaging.

Chemical stress can disrupt our bodies in many ways. It can trigger inflammation in the brain, which is linked to depression and anxiety. It can also interfere with the hormones the body produces to regulate many of its functions.

Researchers estimate that 80% of chronic diseases such as cancer, obesity, diabetes, and heart disease are linked to our diet. Yet, the connection between health and diet in the United States has been ignored for too long.

Fear Not

Chemicals and toxins can be dangerous, but many factors – such as the dose and amount of exposure over time — determine the level of risk. Also, our bodies have the ability to detoxify, adapt, and heal, even while living in challenging environments.

Becoming aware of and understanding the danger of these external threats is important. It will help us make informed choices when shopping for food and other daily-use items. But worrying and regretting poor diet choices can put the body into a fight-or-flight state. This triggers the release of stress hormones, which may be more damaging to our health than the chemicals in our food!

Gratitude triggers the release of hormones that help our bodies relax, detoxify, and heal. So rather than falling victim to fear, choose to be grateful for the people taking action to clean up our food supply.

Made in the USA

Because the chemicals they contain have been shown to cause health problems, some foods made in the US are banned in other countries. However, many food manufacturers in the US create healthier versions of their products so they can sell them in countries with stricter laws and regulations.

The European Union (EU) requires warning labels on most foods containing artificial dyes because they may harm a child's activity and ability to pay attention. Other countries, including Peru, Chile, and Ecuador, require a warning label on foods that contain high amounts of sugar, fat, or calories.

In November 2023, *The Guardian,* a British daily newspaper founded in 1821, reported that Colombia passed a "junk food law" to help reduce the number of lifestyle-related diseases in the country. The law places a 10% tax on junk food to discourage the purchase of unhealthy food. The tax increases to 20% by 2025. The leader of the Colombian advocacy group, Beatriz Champagne, said, "We want to avoid the path of rich industrialized nations, such as the U.S., where diet-linked diseases are a big problem."

Some American-made foods banned in other countries include:

- Instant stuffing and mashed potatoes

- Some American sweet treats (A Google search will tell you which ones.)

- Bread made with potassium bromate

- Products containing high-fructose corn syrup

SAD DAD

The Standard American Diet (**SAD**), also known as the Deadly American Diet (**DAD**), makes people sick.

Gas station snack shops, television commercials, billboards, vending machines, drive-through fast-food restaurants, and convenience food displayed in grocery stores tempt us to satisfy our hunger with food-like products loaded with chemicals and sugars. These foods do not nourish or heal us. Many times, they just leave us wanting more.

Becoming aware of the hidden chemicals and additives in our food supply and understanding the threat they pose to our health is the first step to avoiding danger.

Chapter Fifteen

The Food Industry

Let your food be your medicine,
and let your medicine be your food.
—Hippocrates 460

Obviously, we did not heed the words of Hippocrates. Rather than focus on food as medicine, the food industry focuses on making money. They hire scientists to determine which foods taste good to humans, and then manufacture food-like products that look appealing, taste good, and have a long shelf life. Many of these foods are loaded with sugar, salt, fat, and chemicals to enhance the flavor and texture.

For years, public-health advocates have been pushing to have the FDA remove certain chemicals from the U.S. food supply, and progress is being made.

- In October 2023, California became the first state to ban certain chemicals, including Red Dye No. 3.

- In January 2025, the USFDA followed suit, and announced a national ban on Red Dye No. 3 after it was found to cause cancer in male rats.

- In April 2025, the USFDA, in collaboration with the US Department of Health and Human Services (HHS), announced plans to phase out eight more dyes from the food supply by the end of 2026.

Food factories have until January 2028 to remove Red Dye No.3 from their products. Factory foods, aka "Frankenfoods," that contain Red Dye No.3, include:

- Candies such as candy corn, lollipops, jelly beans, and candy necklaces

- Vegan *meats* including imitation bacon and sausages

- Icings, especially red or pink frostings

- Sausages and hot dogs

- Cotton candy

- Many cereals

Red Dye No. 3 is used by drug companies to give a red color to some prescription drugs, over-the-counter medications, and vitamin supplements.

Medications used to treat symptoms caused by food dyes sometimes contain the very dye that was causing the problem in the first place! Drugs containing Red Dye No. 3 include:

- Some pain relievers

- Some heartburn medications

- Some vitamin gummies for children and adults

- Some cough medicines

In March 2025, top executives from major food companies, including Smucker's, Kellogg's, General Mills, Kraft Heinz, and PepsiCo. met with HHS and expressed a willingness to take steps to improve the health standards of their food products.

Ultra-Processed Foods (UPFs)

Ultra-Processed Foods (UPFs) contain harmful chemicals leading to chronic diseases. Often purchased as a quick and easy way to feed ourselves and our loved ones, UPFs are more processed than other foods.

Additives used to manufacture ultra-processed foods include:

- Artificial colors

- Artificial flavors

- Preservatives to prevent spoilage and extend shelf life

- Trans fats (hydrogenated oils)

- High-Fructose Corn Syrup

Some of the many foods considered to be ultra-processed include:

- Sports drinks (aka "chemical cocktails")

- Soda

- Packaged meat

- Packaged snacks

- Sweetened breakfast cereals

- Meal replacement shakes

- Instant soups

- Flavored yogurt

Not All Processed Foods Are Bad

Used sparingly, small amounts of sugar, or salt added to many processed foods can be tolerated very well by most people. The list of foods that are considered healthy-processed foods include:

- Canned beans and lentils

- Canned fish

- Oatmeal

- Nuts and nut butters

- Frozen vegetables and fruit

- Hummus

- Milk

- Cottage cheese

- Plain yogurt

What You Can Do

Sudden, radical changes to your diet are not recommended because they are hard to maintain, but small changes can have a significant impact. Start with making small changes, such as:

- Exchange sugar and chemical drinks with filtered water.

- Begin reading labels on foods you buy.

- Identify and reduce the amount of UPFs.

The amount of chemicals used in food production can be frightening. The good news is that action is being taken to remove chemicals from our food supply. Understanding the threat and making better choices can improve our health and the health of our loved ones. What is one change you can make in your grocery shopping this week?

Chapter Sixteen
Scientific Studies

Scientific studies provide us with information we can use and need, but we want to make sure the findings of studies include strong evidence, rather than just observations. Also, scientific studies should include a large sample size. A study with just 50 or 100 people may not be reliable, and a single study on a particular food may not be enough to provide the information we need to know. Sometimes scientific studies regarding food can be biased because:

- Some studies are funded by corporations whose products are being studied.

- Some studies rely on self-reporting from the people participating, and the information collected can be inaccurate.

- Some studies, such as finding people who eat a certain food live longer, may not consider other factors of cause-and-effect that could be involved.

- Not all scientific studies are published. Those with findings such as "This food makes you lose weight!" are the ones that get our attention.

- Scientists conducting the studies are human beings who have their own beliefs and biases.

- Experts in statistics say a minimum of 100 participants should be included in a study. Many times, that's not enough data to reach a definite conclusion.

Think for Yourself

In 1987, Lee Iacocca, known for his leadership roles at Ford and Chrysler, addressed the graduating class at Duke University, telling them they needed to learn to think for themselves.

Today, with large corporations deciding what to put in the food we buy, we need to be informed, especially in the face of commercial influences and conflicting data. Social media is filled with people from all walks of life doing their best to influence people with their health advice. But the bottom line is that we need to think for ourselves.

When it comes to protecting and maintaining our health, choosing what to eat is one of the most important decisions we make every day. We need to do what we can to educate ourselves in order to make better choices.

Informed Consent

Informed consent is a term used by health-care providers to ensure that a patient understands what they are agreeing to, what will be done to them, and what risks are involved. Similarly, when it comes to the food we purchase, we should understand the risks and benefits so that we can make the best decision for ourselves and our health.

Scientific studies suggest that the following foods are probably safe, but we each need to decide for ourselves whether to limit certain ones.

Fatty Acids

Fatty acids serve as building blocks of the fats found in our body. They are used to build cell membranes and brain tissue, and some are used to make hormones that support immune function. Fatty acids also play a role in maintaining healthy skin.

There are different types of fatty acids. Some are made in the body, while others are essential — meaning the body cannot produce them and they must be provided through the diet. According to some studies, certain fatty acids in our diet are beneficial, while others — if consumed in excess — are linked to health problems. Here is a summary of what you need to know about them.

Saturated Fatty Acids

Saturated fatty acids come from animal products such as butter, cheese, and red meat. They provide building blocks for our cells, but too much can raise levels of bad cholesterol and increase inflammation. They should be used in moderation.

Unsaturated Fatty Acids

Unsaturated fatty acids are healthy fatty acids that reduce inflammation and improve heart health. There are two types of unsaturated fatty acids:

Monounsaturated fatty acids are found in olive oil, almonds, peanuts, and avocados. They reduce inflammation, improve heart health, and maintain blood sugar levels. They contain Omega-9 fatty acids, which can be produced by the body.

Polyunsaturated fatty acids include Omega-3 and Omega-6, which are essential because they are not produced by the body and must be obtained through the diet.

Omega-3 Fatty Acids

Omega-3 fatty acids are found in fatty fish such as salmon and sardines, as well as walnuts, flaxseeds, and chia seeds. Omega-3 fatty acids can:

- Reduce inflammation
- Improve heart health

- Support brain development and cognitive function

- May help alleviate symptoms of depression, anxiety, and cognitive decline

Omega-6 Fatty Acids

Omega-6 fatty acids are found in seed oils such as corn oil, soybean oil, and sunflower oil. The health benefits of Omega-6 include:

- Maintaining nerves and a healthy brain

- Supporting skin, hair, and eye health

- Regulating hormones

- Helping to lower bad cholesterol

According to studies, the problem with Omega-6 fatty acids is that if they are not consumed in a proper balance with Omega-3 fatty acids, they can promote inflammation.

Omega-6 Dominance

The ideal ratio of Omega-6 to Omega-3 is believed to be 4:1 or lower. Consuming ultra-processed foods high in Omega-6s, and foods from fast-food restaurants that use seed oils for frying, make that ratio nearly impossible to achieve. This may lead to inflammation and chronic diseases.

Recent findings from Weill Cornell Medicine suggest that Omega-6 fatty acids may accelerate the growth of certain aggressive forms of breast cancer. This further highlights the need to rebalance modern Omega-6/Omega-3 intake ratios.

Fast-food restaurants that use oils high in Omega-6 to fry their food have come under scrutiny. Some are beginning to switch from using seed oils to other types that are not high in Omega-6 fatty acids.

Seed Oils

Seed oils include corn oil, sunflower oil, soybean oil, and canola oil. Seed oils contain Omega-6 fatty acids, which may be harmful to our health if not enough Omega-3 fatty acids are consumed to achieve a proper ratio.

Instead of seed oils, plant-based oils such as olive oil and avocado oil, which contain a better ratio of Omega-3 fatty acids, are often recommended.

What You Can Do

- Read food labels and limit use of seed oils.

- Replace seed oils with olive oil or avocado oil.

- Include fatty fish such as salmon and sardines in your diet.

- Add walnuts, flax seeds, and chia seeds to your diet.

- Limit the amount of butter, cheese, and red meat.

Hogwash!

That Omega-6 fatty acids are bad for you is controversial.

The Harvard Newsletter published a story in April 2019 defending the reputation of Omega-6 fatty acids. They explained how Omega-6 fatty acids can lower harmful LDL cholesterol, boost good HDL cholesterol, and improve the body's use of insulin to keep blood sugar levels in check. They admit that the problem with Omega-6 is it can be converted into a substance that promotes inflammation and blood clotting, but it can also be converted to a substance that fights inflammation!

The newsletter says experts suggesting we limit the amount of Omega-6 fatty acids to improve the ratio of Omega-3 to Omega-6 is considered by The American Heart Association to be hogwash because Omega-6 fatty acids are good for the heart.

Both Omega-3 and Omega-6 fatty acids are essential. Our body cannot make them. We must get them from the foods we eat. According to the report, the best way to improve the ratio is to eat more Omega-3s, not fewer Omega-6s.

Choosing a Diet

In the past, many extreme fad diets that promised to improve health turned out to be quite harmful. From the tapeworm diet in the early 1900s, which promised weight loss, to the sleeping beauty diet in the 1960s, which involved taking sedatives to sleep rather than eat, many fad diets have come — and thankfully, gone.

When it comes to choosing which diet to follow, the amount of misinformation available makes choosing a diet confusing and overwhelming.

Some popular diets today include:

- **Carnivore Diet** – All animal products.

- **Veganism** – No animal products.

- **Paleo Diet** – Animal and plant products, but avoiding grains, beans, dairy products and seed oils

- **The Ketogenic Diet** – low-carb/no-carb, high-fat diet of meat, high-fat dairy, healthy oils, low-carb vegetables, but no grains, sugars, starchy veggies, and no fruit except for a small number of berries.

- **Intermittent Fasting** – an eating pattern that restricts the time you are allowed to eat rather than what you are allowed to eat. The most popular is fasting for 16 hours and limiting eating to an eight-hour window.

- **OMAD** – a variation of intermittent fasting that allows one meal a day.

- **Intuitive Eating** – Listening to your body and choosing foods that sound good to you.

- **The Mediterranean Diet** - Backed by decades of research, The Mediterranean Diet has been linked to a longer life, lower heart disease, and better brain health.

A Common-Sense Diet

The Mediterranean Diet is high in fruits, vegetables, whole grains, and healthy fats such as olive oil and nuts. It includes fish, dairy, chicken, and eggs. It is low in processed foods and red meat. Compared to other diets, the Mediterranean Diet seems like a good choice, especially if you are looking for a common-sense diet.

Everyone is different, and no single diet works for all. However, avoiding ultra-processed foods and choosing whole or minimally-processed foods should be the foundation of any healthy eating plan.

Some people do well on a simple, balanced diet, avoiding harmful ingredients, and enjoying everything in moderation. When it comes to planning a personalized diet to support overall health, a nutritional therapist can help. Those with specific health conditions may want to find a certified functional medicine professional to help plan a diet that addresses your concerns.

There are professional directories available online to help locate a certified practitioner. From there you can check their website, read Google reviews, and book a consultation (sometimes free) to discuss your concerns.

The following directories are a good place to start:

Institute for Functional Medicine (IFM)
Certified Practitioners:
www.ifm.org

Nutritional Therapy Association (NTA) Practitioners:
www.nutritionaltherapy.com

Academy of Nutrition and Dietetics includes registered dieticians who specialize in functional medicine. www.eatright.org

Scheduling a checkup with your healthcare provider before starting a new diet is highly recommended.

The Takeaway

Keeping an open mind when reading scientific studies allows you to gain valuable insights and information. Be aware of potential biases that may have influenced the findings.

Chapter Seventeen

What's in Your Kitchen?

As part of my research for this section, I decided to inspect my kitchen. I wanted to find out if there are harmful ingredients in the food I buy at the grocery store each week.

When I opened the cupboard, the first thing I inspected was a can of organic black beans. I was pleased to see it had only three ingredients: organic black beans, water, and salt. That's good, I thought, placing the can back into the cupboard.

Then I picked up a bag of organic basmati rice, but there was no ingredient list. At first, I thought that was odd, maybe even illegal, but then I realized, it's only rice! Just rice, nothing else. Just like it says on the bag.

The same thing with honey. No ingredient list. Just honey!

Then I picked up a can of tuna fish. Again, just three ingredients: tuna, water, and salt.

Also, in my cupboard was a package of cereal bars marketed as a healthy snack, but the ingredient list included many chemicals I didn't recognize or couldn't pronounce.

I thought about donating the box to the local food pantry, but instead, I tossed it into the trash. I would rather donate healthy food to people struggling to feed themselves and their families.

Next, I turned my attention to the refrigerator. I was pleased to see my organic almond butter, packaged organic lettuce, and arugula all had only one ingredient.

One-ingredient food suddenly became my favorite foods.

Protein Powder

When I looked at the protein powder I use to make a shake every day, I saw that it contained "natural flavors" and other ingredients I didn't recognize or couldn't pronounce. This was disappointing and I asked Google about it.

"Natural flavors" add flavor rather than nutritional value to food. The FDA does not always review the specific ingredients in natural flavorings. Some reports say "natural flavors" contain chemical colors, preservatives, solvents, and emulsifiers. To my dismay, I discovered protein powders are considered an ultra-processed food, and some may contain lead. How did I not know this? Now what?

I began looking at the labels of various protein powders and found one that contained the least amount of ingredients. The fact that I add fruit or vegetables to my protein shakes makes it acceptable for now. I am incorporating other forms of protein into my diet rather than depending so heavily on protein powder.

Food as Fuel

I began thinking of food as fuel when I worked as a massage therapist at a salon on Worth Avenue in Palm Beach. During that time in my life, I was burning the candle at both ends. I was working as a massage therapist during the day and attending college at night to earn the math and science credits I needed to get into chiropractic college.

Giving hour-long massages all day long was hard work. It required a lot of energy. I remember going into the break room one day, feeling hungry and tired and wondering how I would be able to do another four massages that day. As I ate my lunch (probably a peanut butter and jelly sandwich on whole-wheat bread) I felt my energy returning, and I remember thinking, "Food is fuel."

Thinking of food as fuel makes it easier to choose high-nutrient options, but food is more than fuel — it's also a natural part of human culture, community, and finding joy in the simple pleasures of life. Mindfully enjoying food can benefit both our emotional and physical health.

Recreational Eating

Pleasure and enjoyment play a significant role in our sense of well-being, so it's important not to feel guilty when enjoying the foods we like. It's all about moderation and mindfulness. Recreational eating is a natural part of human culture and can be part of a healthy lifestyle. Enjoying food with others can reduce stress and build social connections.

Practicing portion control, planning ahead by eating lighter during the day, and focusing on connecting with others rather than just the food, are good ways to make recreational eating part of a healthy lifestyle.

The dangers of recreational eating include overeating to cope with stress, feeling guilty when enjoying an occasional treat, and ignoring natural body cues of hunger and fullness. Practicing mindfulness when eating helps prevent these problems.

Coffee

Some studies say coffee is bad for you and others say it's good for you. But when it comes to studies about coffee, I don't care — I'm not giving it up!

Jerry Seinfeld probably agrees. During an appearance on the Jimmy Fallon show, Seinfeld said,

"Coffee is the most important part of a human's life. It's the only thing that is 100 percent on your side. Every day, every cup, come on, let's go, we can do this!"

Another quote that supports my morning cup of coffee is:

> *Give me coffee to change the things I can,*
> *and a visit to the beach to change*
> *the things I cannot.*

If coffee is bad for me, I will just consider it part of my 20 percent.

The 80/20 Rule

We are only human, so rather than be too hard on yourself, you can use the 80/20 rule. Eating for health 80 percent of the time, and allowing yourself to relax about 20 percent of the time, is a good starting point for improving your diet and overall well-being. By eliminating harmful foods from your diet, you will reduce your exposure to substances that can negatively affect your health.

What You Can Do

- Perform a kitchen audit and get rid of the ultra-processed foods you can do without.

- Make a shopping list of healthy foods and stick to it.

- Keep a diet diary. Writing down "two donuts at the drive-thru on the way to work" makes for a good wake-up call.

Improving your diet by making better choices at the grocery store doesn't require a lot of money. In fact, it can save you money. Highly-processed and packaged foods are more costly than simple ingredients that can be used to make meals at home.

Eating Healthy on a Budget

It's important to recognize that not everyone has equal access to organic groceries. But awareness is free. Even the smallest adjustments, such as reading a label, choosing water over soda, or cooking one more meal at home each week, can make a meaningful difference.

Eating healthy on a tight budget is possible. A good first step is to take a look at what you have in your kitchen. From there, create a weekly meal plan, then make a shopping list for items you need to buy. Sticking to a list helps avoid unnecessary spending.

Learning to prepare simple meals at home, rather than relying on fast food and ultra-processed products, can be healthier and more cost-effective.

One-Pot Meals

Learning to prepare one-pot meals such as stews, chili, and stir-fries can be a rewarding and delicious way to begin cooking at home. All you need to get started is a pot, a knife, a cutting board, and a spoon. A pot of rice and beans cooked at home can be both satisfying and delicious. You can enhance your cooking with a variety of spices that add rich, delicious flavors.

Other simple recipes can be made in batches and frozen for easy, budget-friendly meals later. To learn more about how to begin cooking at home, free cooking classes and workshops are sometimes offered by food banks, churches, and local community centers.

Many YouTube channels show how easy it is for beginners to make simple, three-ingredient recipes the family will enjoy.

YouTube University

Anyone with access to a smart phone or computer can tune into YouTube and find videos to teach you how to cook simple, healthy meals. Finding a channel you like is easy.

For example, in the search bar, I typed "Healthy three-minute meals on a budget for people who don't have time or know how to cook." Some of the results include short videos such as:

- Twenty healthy meals for $30

- Five easy and healthy one-pot meals

- Healthy meals on a budget

- Cheap and healthy meals for the week in one hour

- Ultra easy healthy meals, but cheaper

Rather than doomscrolling or wasting time on Facebook or other apps, spend a few minutes each day attending cooking classes on YouTube University and find yourself a cooking coach… for free!

The thing about YouTube is that when you search for a topic, the YouTube algorithm begins sending you similar videos. Before you know it, you will be discovering other channels that meet your needs for information.

I enjoy watching a fellow who came across my YouTube feed who makes healthy meals in three minutes or less, which really appealed to me. Lately, he's been featuring 30-second healthy snacks! I find his videos to be very informative and very entertaining.

What You Can Do

Start where you are, use what you have, and take one step at a time toward a healthier diet.

- Buy beans, rice, oats, lentils, eggs, and frozen vegetables.

- Buy canned tuna and sardines.

- Don't waste money on processed snacks.

- Drink water instead of soda.

Chapter Eighteen

It's Never Too Late

The good news is that it's never too late. Starting today, you can begin reducing — or better yet, eliminating — junk food from your diet.

Recently, I saw a patient for the first time in three months. When I first saw him about a year ago, he was suffering from chronic pain and discomfort from an old injury. He was on a call-as-needed basis. When I saw him recently, I was pleasantly surprised by how much better he looked and how much better he said he felt.

"I decided to become proactive in my health," he said.

He told me he cleaned up his diet, lost 15 pounds, quit eating junk food, and stopped drinking alcohol.

"As I started to feel better, I became more inspired to take better care of my health," he said. "You get to a point in life where you have to make the decision to change your ways."

Transmutation – An Interesting Idea

In 1925, French chemist C. Louis Kervran proposed the controversial idea of transmutation, suggesting that the human body may be able to convert one element into another to meet its nutritional needs. He based his theory on the observation that shellfish can create a new shell in water that contains no calcium.

He also questioned how chickens could produce egg-shells composed of calcium carbonate when they were fed oats. He explained it by saying that oats must be combined with hydrogen to produce calcium.

His theory lacks mainstream scientific validation. It earned him an Ig Nobel Prize, a satirical award that makes people first laugh, and then think.

Some alternative medicine practitioners explore its potential implications, and I find the idea of transmutation to be intriguing. Like many far-out ideas I come across in an effort to learn everything I can about health and healing, I think to myself, "Why not? Can't hurt, might help." ☺

When it comes to Kervran's theory, it can't hurt and it might help, so while eating, I sometimes like to think and say, "Everything I eat makes me strong and healthy."

Feeling good about the food we are eating improves our body's ability to assimilate nutrients and eliminate waste products from our bodies. Feeling fear that the food we are eating might make us sick triggers the stress response, the opposite of where we need to be when we eat.

Rest and Digest

Suppose our stress response is activated, and we are in survival mode while eating. During the fight-or-flight response, blood is diverted from our digestive system to our muscles. In that case, our body cannot digest food properly.

When we eat, we should be in rest-and-digest mode so our body can properly assimilate the nutrients. Taking a moment before eating or drinking to allow our body to shift gears from fight-or-flight to rest-and-digest helps us absorb nutrients from our food more effectively.

Giving Thanks

Feeling grateful for our food puts us into rest-and-digest mode. This prepares our body to begin the process of digestion, which starts in the mouth. As we mindfully chew our food, salivary glands release digestive enzymes that mix with it. Chewing our food paves the way for a smooth journey to our stomach and through our gut.

Chewing our food is important, but we may not have to be as extreme as the popular chewing method promoted by Horace Fletcher back in the 1900s. The idea of Fletcherism was to chew each bite of food up to 100 times until it became completely liquid before swallowing. He believed doing so would improve digestion, and people would naturally eat less. He also said we should eat only when hungry, not out of habit, and never eat when upset or angry.

There is no evidence that spending so much time chewing food leads to better digestion, but we could all probably slow down a little and practice mindful eating. After all, we are busy humans, not cows, who have the time to spend 8 hours a day chewing their cud. Besides, that could add up to 30-40,000 jaw movements a day, a lot of extra work for our temporomandibular (TMJ) jaw joints!

The Takeaway

You are what you eat. You are not junk so don't eat junk. Choose foods that heal you, not harm you.

Chapter Nineteen
Our Digestive Tube

Our gut can be thought of as a hollow tube with openings at each end. At one end is the mouth; at the other end, the anus. Even though it runs through the center of our body, this hollow passageway is technically considered outside our body. It is lined with a permeable membrane made of specialized cells that allow nutrients, liquids and gas to pass through. This muscular tube is about 30 feet long and includes:

- Our mouth secretes digestive enzymes and produces more along the way.

- The stomach is 10 inches long when empty, but expands.

- The small intestine is 22 feet long. It winds back and forth, absorbing nutrients.

- The large intestine is five to six feet long, circles the abdomen, absorbs water, and forms a solid stool.

- The rectum is for temporary storage.

- The anus eliminates waste,

Our Second Brain

With more than 100 million nerve cells embedded in the walls of our gut, scientists refer to this area of our bodies as our second brain. This second brain works independently of the brain in our head to control the automatic process of digestion.

This second brain is controlled by the vagus nerve, which receives information from the senses and sends signals to the brain, creating emotional and physical reactions to circumstances. These physical sensations are commonly referred to as gut instincts, intuition, sixth sense, or a hunch.

Trusting your gut is often advised to those seeking answers to their questions. For instance, in one of her television programs, Suze Orman, financial consultant to the masses, advised a woman who was trying to make a decision to listen to her gut. The woman had called into Orman's show, saying her boyfriend wanted her to sell her house, quit her job, and move into his rented home.

"What does your gut tell you?" asked an incredulous Orman, furrowing her brow and cocking her head at the television camera so viewers could see her skepticism.

Hearing this woman's story, my first thought was that she was probably under the influence of oxytocin. Oxytocin is a hormone released during intimate contact.

It makes women want to create and maintain emotional bonds. That young woman was hoping to preserve a bond with her boyfriend, even at the risk of financial ruin. I listened intently, waiting for the woman's reply.

"My gut tells me not to do it," said the woman sheepishly.

Orman smiled a big, victorious smile. "Girlfriend," she said, pointing her index finger toward the camera, "you are wise to listen to your gut."

Our subconscious mind is constantly processing information and sending chemical messengers to our conscious brain via the vagus nerve. We need to pay attention to sensations in our abdomen. These gut feelings can alert us to potential danger, help us make good decisions, and affirm that a decision was correct through the calm feeling that follows a wise choice.

Some say the subconscious mind is our connection to God or our higher self, but no one knows for sure. We need to be careful though, because gut feelings can be influenced by fear and wishful thinking. Still, listening to our gut can be helpful at times.

Gut-Brain Axis

The brain in our head and the brain in our gut communicate via the vagus nerve. Scientists are only beginning to understand how significant this relationship may be. Some interesting findings regarding the influence of the gut-brain axis include:

- About 90 percent of the happy hormone, serotonin, is produced in the gut.

- Levels of inflammation in the gut are related to brain health.

For instance, research teams in France are developing a theory that Parkinson's disease may start in the gut and make its way to the brain.

Digestive disturbances in Parkinson's patients can begin many years before the disease is diagnosed. Researchers have found that biopsies of nerve cells in the gut of Parkinson's patients show similar disturbances to those found in nerve cells in the brain. They hope early detection — years before neurological symptoms appear — can lead to early intervention and treatment.

Researchers are also studying the relationship between Alzheimer's disease and the gut-brain axis. A 2023 study suggests inflammation could be the cause, as patients with Alzheimer's disease have high levels of gut inflammation. Animal studies have demonstrated that Alzheimer's disease can be transmitted to young mice through the transfer of microbiome, which includes gut bacteria.

We all have different types of microbiomes, which could explain why different diets work for different people. Research involving the transfer of microbiomes from one person to another is currently under way.

Our Gut Bacteria

Our body contains more bacteria cells than human cells, and most of them live in our colon. No one knows for sure, but according to an article published in the Harvard Gazette, microbiologists say the human body has about 30 trillion human cells and 39 trillion bacteria.

The gut bacteria, referred to as our gut microbiome, include bacteria, viruses, and fungi. These require a microscope to see. The bacteria in our gut play an important role in regulating inflammation. They do this in several different ways:

- They fight off harmful microbes.

- They produce vitamins.

- They produce serotonin and dopamine that affect our mood in positive ways.

- They produce proteins to strengthen the walls of our digestive tube.

- They produce beneficial short-chain beneficial fatty acids from the fermented fiber we eat.

- They help regulate our metabolism.

A diet high in processed foods, excessive sugar, insufficient fiber, chronic stress, lack of sleep, and too much alcohol have been linked to disrupting the balance of good and bad gut bacteria. Maintaining a healthy balance between these bacteria is important, as an imbalance can lead to autoimmune diseases, nutritional deficiencies, and digestive diseases such as cancer.

The good news is that our gut is the most highly regenerative organ in our body. Amazingly, it regenerates its lining every 5-7 days, even while enduring the stress of digesting food, assimilating nutrients, and eliminating waste from our body.

Prebiotics

Prebiotics improve the balance between the good and bad bacteria in our gut by feeding the good bacteria.

Unlike live bacteria found in probiotics, prebiotics are a type of fiber found in plant foods. Prebiotics are broken down by our microbiome and form short-chain fatty acids. These fatty acids help with digestion, reduce inflammation, and strengthen the immune system.

Foods that contain prebiotics contain fiber and starch, such as fruits and vegetables. Some of the best prebiotic foods include:

- Garlic, onions, and leeks

- Asparagus

- Jerusalem Artichokes

- Bananas – especially unripe green ones.

- Apples

- Berries

- Oats

- Lentils and chickpeas

- Flaxseeds and chia seeds

Probiotics

Probiotics are live microorganisms that can be consumed to improve gut health. Some common probiotic microorganisms are lactobacillus, bifidobacterium, and bacillus.

Probiotics can help improve digestion, support skin health, and prevent infections. They are found in foods such as yogurt, kefir, and kimchi. Probiotics can also be taken as dietary supplements.

Antibiotics

Antibiotics are necessary to fight infections, but they can kill both good and bad bacteria. That is why doctors often recommend taking a probiotic to help restore balance to the microbiome. Depending on the situation, doctors may recommend probiotics be taken during or after the antibiotic treatment.

Our gut works hard for us, so we should do all we can to make the job of our friendly bacteria a little easier. By the way, our friendly bacteria may be smarter than we think. Just ask your mitochondria — they will tell you all about it.

Mitochondria

Mitochondria are known as the power house of our cells because they are involved in the process of creating energy from the food we eat. There are thousands of mitochondria inside each cell, but what's especially interesting is the widely accepted theory that they were once free-living bacteria.

Mitochondria, formerly known as bacteria, did a good job creating energy from the food we eat. They were promoted and are now recognized as an important component of human cells.

Scientists believe mitochondria used to be a bacterium because they exhibit traits similar to bacteria:

- They reproduce by dividing.

- They have a membrane and a cell wall.

- They have their own genetic material and …

- They communicate with other mitochondria! (But nobody knows what they are saying about us.)

Happy Liver Day!

April 19th is World Liver Day. The aim of that day is to highlight the importance of the liver and inform people about how they can keep it healthy. When it comes to maintaining health and preventing illness, the liver is not as popular as the heart and brain, but the liver is just as important. We cannot live without it.

An important organ in the digestive process, the liver could be compared to the oil filter in a car. Once the intestines have finished digesting and absorbing nutrients from the food we eat, blood leaves through tiny vessels in the intestinal wall and flows to a vein that leads to the liver.

The liver processes more than a quart of blood per minute, which adds up to more than 500 gallons a day. It filters out toxins, absorbs and stores nutrients, then sends the blood to a vein that carries it back to the heart to be oxygenated before circulating through the body.

The liver produces bile, which is stored in the gallbladder. When we eat fat, the gallbladder releases a small amount of bile into the small intestine to help break it down as it moves through the digestive tract.

Our liver is located on the right side of our body, just beneath the last rib of our rib cage. It is sometimes referred to as the largest organ in the body. That's not true. The skin, which is also an organ, is the largest organ of the body. But the liver is pretty big. In the average adult, the liver weighs about three and a half pounds.

When the liver becomes sick, it can become inflamed, as in hepatitis, or it can become scarred and fibrous, a condition known as cirrhosis. Most people associate cirrhosis of the liver with excessive alcohol, but taking too many medications can also cause a form of cirrhosis called chemical cirrhosis.

Your mouth is the gateway to your gut. Your gut is your gateway to health. The gut can be thought of as the body's sewer system, eliminating waste products -including toxins, after nutrients are absorbed from food. Take care of your gut, and your gut will take care of you.

Chapter Twenty

Environmental Toxins

What doesn't kill you makes you stronger.
—Fredrich Nietzsche

In 1888, Nietzsche wrote this in his book. His famous quote is frequently used when discussing how humans can survive and thrive during times of adversity. His quote provides a glimmer of hope to those who are concerned about the threat of environmental toxins to our health.

The word *hormesis* is a term used in biology to describe how small amounts of toxins can trigger the cells of our body to adapt, repair, and become more resilient. Of course, there is a limit to the amount of toxins that can be tolerated, but hormesis demonstrates our body's ability to adapt.

Also, our bodies have built-in mechanisms for detoxi-fication. For instance:

- The liver filters 500 gallons of blood each day, breaking down toxins and making them easy to excrete.

- The kidneys filter 50 gallons of blood each day and do a great job neutralizing and excreting toxic substances from our body.

- The lungs process and expel toxins (which is how breathalyzers detect alcohol).

- The skin eliminates toxins through sweat glands.

- The gut eliminates toxins through bowel movements.

- The immune system identifies and neutralizes toxins.

There is a limit to the amount of toxins our body can process, but there are many things we can do to assist our body's detoxification systems, including:

- Hydrate with filtered water.

- Practice deep breathing.

- Exercise and sweat.

- Eat fiber-rich foods.

- Get enough sleep.

- Minimize toxic intake.

Not everyone who comes into contact with chemicals and environmental toxins becomes sick from them.

Staying healthy involves both the constitution and the condition of the body.

Constitution vs. Condition

The constitution of a body refers to its inherited or innate ability to prevent and fight disease. The constitution is determined by genetics, physical structure, and the body's ability to manage chemical processes responsible for assimilating nutrients, eliminating wastes, and making repairs.

Someone with a delicate constitution may need to be more careful in their efforts to stay healthy. Those with a robust constitution may be able to tolerate more abuse before breaking down.

The condition of the body is the result of the things we do to take care of our health. Managing emotional stress, controlling our chemical input, and how we care for our physical body all contribute to the condition of the body.

Epigenetics

Genes are the gun,
but the environment is the trigger

Some people with a history of disease in their family believe it is their fate to inherit that disease, but that's not true.

Epigenetics is the study of how genes in our genetic material can be regulated. This means having a genetic predisposition to certain disease is not necessarily your destiny.

Regulating our gene expression can be accomplished by taking steps to regulate how our body responds to stress.

Understanding the Threat

The threat from chemical and environmental toxins makes planet Earth seem like a dangerous place to live. But don't panic. Freaking out about the effect of environmental toxins on our health causes the release of adrenaline and cortisol and makes matters worse. Practice Navy SEAL breathing, and keep reading; there are many things we can do to lessen external threats.

Understanding the dangers of environmental toxins will empower us to make informed choices for keeping our bodies in good condition, regardless of our constitution. The following chapters are designed to be an introduction to environmental toxins. Included are many simple things we can do to reduce the threat.

A Good Resource

If you want or need more in-depth information about environmental toxins and chemicals, I recommend the book *Fatal Conveniences* by Darin Olien. Like many people, Olien's father suffered from chemical sensitivities and needed to avoid chemicals.

In his book, Olien goes into great depth regarding chemicals in personal-care products, household products, foods and beverages, and even clothing. In his book, he lists many sources for buying products that don't contain harmful substances.

One Word: Plastics

In 1967, the movie *The Graduate* had a scene where the young graduate, Benjamin Braddock, received advice from his father's friend, Mr. McGuire.

"Just one word…Plastics. There's a great future in plastics," said Mr. McGuire, implying that plastic was the path to financial success.

Obviously, a lot of people took that path, because current estimates suggest that more than nine billion tons of plastic have been produced since the 1950s. Plastic is in just about everything, including food, sea life, soil, drinking water, and the tissues and organs of our bodies.

Plastic is a chemical made from a process involving the use of oil and natural gas. Various chemicals are then added to give plastics characteristics such as flexibility, waterproofing, or rigidity, depending upon the type of plastic products being manufactured.

Microplastics

Microplastics are tiny pieces of plastic, about the size of a sesame seed or smaller. There are two types of microplastics.

One type is manufactured as *microbeads* and added to products — from cosmetics to toothpaste — to create texture and benefits. Microbeads were used in products that exfoliate the skin, making it smoother and softer. The use of microbeads in products made in the United States has been banned since 2015. Some products made in European countries are allowed to stay on the market through 2035. Google can help you find out if the products you use contain microbeads.

The other type of microplastics results from plastic bottles, bags, containers, and other plastic items that break down over time. Microplastics are found everywhere, from drinking water to soil to synthetic clothing. Studies are showing a link to health problems, including lung inflammation and heart disease. Studies published in *Brain Medicine* suggest microplastics may contribute to mental-health issues.

Research conducted between 2016 and 2024 at the University of New Mexico found that human brains contain plastic. Some were found to contain an amount of plastic equivalent to that in a plastic spoon! Cadavers diagnosed with dementia had ten times the amount of plastic than those who didn't.

Environmental toxins and chemicals added to our food can interfere with the trillions of chemical processes occurring in our body every second. These processes are controlled by our hormones. Many chemicals and toxins are believed to be hormone disruptors. The common abbreviation for hormone disruptors is EDC, which stands for endocrine-disrupting chemicals.

Hormones

Hormones are the body's chemical messengers. They are released by various glands and regulate many different functions. Several glands in the body produce hormones that control various bodily functions.

- The thyroid gland, located in the front of the neck, produces hormones that regulate energy production.

- The adrenal glands, located on top of the kidneys, produce stress hormones, including adrenaline and cortisol.

- The pancreas, located behind the stomach, produces hormones, including insulin to regulate blood-sugar levels.

- The ovaries in females produce sex hormones, including estrogen and progesterone.

- The testes in males produce testosterone.

Microplastics often contain chemicals that have been linked to disrupt the hormonal system of the body. This may lead to reproductive and developmental issues. Listed below are environmental toxins that have been linked to hormonal disturbances.

Phthalates (pronounced THAL-ates)

Phthalates are common chemicals used to make plastics more flexible and durable. They are found in everyday products such as toys, air fresheners, and any household product with artificial fragrances. They are also found in vinyl flooring and some cosmetics.

Some phthalates are no longer allowed in children's toys, pacifiers, or baby bottles, but others are still permitted in plastics used for food storage. Most people have measurable levels of phthalates in their bodies. Understanding what they are and where they are found can help you make better choices and avoid adding more.

Warning labels or information about the safety of chemicals used in plastic containers is not legally required. Still, many plastic manufacturers mark their products with a number from one to seven inside a triangle for the purpose of recycling.

The numbers also identify the type of resin used in producing the plastic, but they don't tell you what the plastic contains, whether it's microwave- or dishwasher-safe, or how much it can leach chemicals into your food.

Some plastic food containers are safer than others. It is best to limit their use, especially for foods that can increase chemical leaching such as hot, spicy, or fatty foods.

Phthalates are linked to hormonal disturbances, especially testosterone and estrogen. Boys exposed to phthalates in the womb may be born with feminization of genitalia or undescended testicles. Studies have linked phthalates to an increase in asthma, eczema, and other health disorders in children.

What You Can Do

- If possible, avoid plastic food containers. Use glass, stainless steel, or silicone instead.

- Never microwave food in plastic.

- Use wooden rather than plastic cutting boards.

- Choose fragrance-free or naturally scented products.

- Avoid plastic toys not labelled as phthalate-free.

BPA -Bisphenol A

BPA is a chemical used in making certain plastics. It is found in plastic containers, especially those marked with the number seven.

Chemicals used to coat cans and containers are not usually disclosed, but companies can voluntarily label the plastic as BPA-free for educated consumers.

BPA is a hormone disruptor. Studies indicate that BPA can mimic and interfere with estrogen and may cause infertility, early puberty, and other health problems.

What You Can Do

- Use glass, stainless steel, or plastic items certified BPA-free. Look for BPA-free canned items.

- Drink filtered water.

- BPAs are used to coat thermal paper receipts, so whenever possible, decline paper receipts.

PFAs – Polyfluoroalkyl Substances

PFAs are chemicals discovered in the 1940s by a chemist working for DuPont. He was looking to create a refrigerant but instead developed a substance resistant to water and grease. This led to the use of Teflon in cookware. PFAs are known as "forever chemicals" because they do not break down easily in the human body or the environment.

From nonstick cookware and water-repellent clothing, to fast-food wrappers, microwave popcorn bags, thermal paper receipts, stain-resistant furniture and carpets, PFAs are everywhere. Almost everyone has PFAs in their blood, and because these chemicals remain in the body for years, frequent exposure can become significant.

Research has linked PFAs to many health conditions, including thyroid disease, hormone disruptions, developmental problems in children, and some cancers, including kidney and testicular.

What You Can Do

- Avoid non-stick cookware. Use stainless steel, ceramic, or cast iron instead.

- Limit exposure to fast-food wrappers.

- Look for product labels that say PFAS-free or PFDA-free.

- Drink filtered water.

NOTE: When I found out most dental floss is coated with PFAs, I looked online and found some that contain no PFAs. Other common items that contain PFAs include tea bags, toothbrushes, and toilet paper.

Pesticides

The Environmental Protection Agency (EPA) has registered more than 25,000 pesticides for use in the United States, including 600 that are registered for use by the food industry. The EPA establishes the allowable amount of pesticide residue to help keep our food safe. Unless they are certified USDA organic, farmers use pesticides to kill insects, weeds, fungi, and rodents when growing their crops.

Pesticides are designed to kill living organisms. Residues can contaminate water and soil and can be found in the food we buy. Using too much can make pests resistant, requiring even more poison to kill them.

Long-term effects include hormone disruption, as well as reproductive and developmental issues. They are also harmful to bees.

What You Can Do

- Wash fruits and vegetables, especially high-residue foods such as strawberries and spinach.

- Remove outer leaves of lettuce and cabbage.

- Support local farms that limit the use of pesticides.

- Limit use of lawn and garden pesticides at home.

Glyphosate

Glyphosate is the active ingredient in Roundup, and has become the most widely used weed killer in the United States. It is used in agriculture, especially by farmers who grow genetically modified crops (GMOs) such as corn, soy, canola, and sugar beets, because these GMOs are resistant to it. They can spray the crops to kill the weeds, but the GMOs survive.

The ongoing debate over the safety of glyphosate is intense. In 2015, The World Health Organization's (WHO) cancer agency said that glyphosate is a probable human carcinogen, although those claims are being denied.

Studies have linked long-term exposure to glyphosate to farm workers who developed non-Hodgkin's lymphoma. Emerging evidence shows possible links to many other health conditions. But unlike DDT, an insecticide that was banned for use in the U.S. by the EPA on December 31, 1972, glyphosate is still widely used today.

The questions of whether or not glyphosate is a threat to our health has yet to be settled. In the meantime, there are things you can do to limit your exposure.

What You Can Do

- Wash fruits and vegetables before eating them.

- Choose organic and non-GMO foods when possible.

- Use a water filter that can remove glyphosate.

- Avoid using herbicides on your lawn. Learn about natural weed control.

The Environmental Working Group created two lists to educate consumers regarding the amount of pesticide residues in certain foods. Each year, they analyze data from the FDA and create lists to help consumers limit their exposure to pesticides in fruits and vegetables. They call one list the "Dirty Dozen" and the other the "Clean Fifteen."

Note: Although the Environmental Working Group calls some fruits and vegetables the "Dirty Dozen," they also say that a diet high in fruits and vegetables is important for maintaining good health. As in anything, moderation is the key. Doing the best we can do is the best we can do.

The Dirty Dozen

The 2025 version of the "Dirty Dozen" includes foods with the highest residue of pesticides. Buy organic if possible, or wash well.

- Strawberries

- Spinach

- Kale, collard and mustard greens

- Grapes

- Peaches

- Cherries

- Nectarines

- Pears

- Apples

- Blackberries

- Blueberries

- Potatoes

The Clean Fifteen

It's safer to buy organic, but the following "Clean Fifteen" were found to have the lowest pesticide residues.

- Pineapples

- Sweet corn

- Avocados

- Papaya

- Onions

- Sweet Peas (frozen)

- Asparagus

- Cabbage

- Watermelon

- Cauliflower

- Bananas

- Mangoes

- Carrots

- Mushrooms

- Kiwi

How to Wash Vegetables

Studies show that adding one teaspoon of baking soda to two cups of water and soaking produce for fifteen minutes removes more pesticides than plain water or vinegar. Use cold water, because hot water can cause pesticides to be absorbed deeper into the produce. Avoid using soaps or detergents that are not approved for use on produce.

After soaking, scrub firm produce, such as cucumbers and apples, with a vegetable brush or your hands. For leafy greens, swish them in the baking soda and water to remove dirt and residue and then rinse well under running water. Berries, mushrooms, and other delicate produce should only be soaked for about five minutes and then rinsed well in a colander.

Every small change you make to reduce your exposure to environmental toxins is a powerful act of self-care for yourself, your loved ones, and future generations.

The next chapter will explain how our body responds to chemical threats with a process known as "inflammation." Understanding the body's response to external attacks will help inspire us to take steps to reduce the danger.

Chapter Twenty-One

Inflammation

Studies indicate more than 35 percent of Americans suffer from chronic inflammation in their body. Inflammation has been linked to most chronic diseases, including heart disease, diabetes, and cancer.

Inflammation is a response by our immune system that causes redness and swelling. It can be acute, such as the body's temporary reaction to an injury, or it can become chronic.

Chronic inflammation is caused by environmental toxins, chemicals, and stress hormones. Inflammation can affect different parts of our body and cause many different health problems. Symptoms of chronic inflammation include body aches, fatigue, frequent infections, and digestive issues.

An occasional bag of chips won't destroy your health, but a continuous diet of high-chemical foods, excessive amounts of sugar, and excessive exposure to environmental toxins can lead to chronic diseases in the following ways:

- Inflammation damages the joints and skin, leading to conditions such as arthritis and psoriasis.

- Inflammation of the blood vessels causes hardening of the arteries, which can lead to heart attacks and strokes.

- Inflammation makes it more difficult for cells to use glucose, which can lead to high blood-sugar levels and Type II diabetes.

- Inflammation can damage our genetic material, which can lead to abnormal cell formation, as seen in cancer.

- Inflammation damages the cells of the brain and nervous system, which can lead to the buildup of toxic proteins seen in Alzheimer's and other neurological diseases.

- Inflammation damages the lining of the gut, which can lead to digestive disorders.

How to Reduce Inflammation

- **Diet** – Avoid or limit processed foods and alcohol. Eat more fatty fish, such as salmon and sardines, and increase your intake of fruits and vegetables.

- **Consider supplements** – fish oil, vitamin D, and curcumin (from turmeric).

- **Exercise** – Aim for 30 minutes of daily exercise, such as walking or cycling, but avoid overtraining because too much exercise can increase inflammation.

- **Relax** – Chronic stress raises cortisol, which increases inflammation. Use techniques in Section One to manage stress.

- **Hydration** – Divide your weight in half and drink that number of ounces of water each day. Everyone is different and lifestyle must be considered. Some people need more water than others.

- **Sleep** – Aim for seven to nine hours each night

- **Support Gut Health** – The bacteria in our gut regulate inflammation. Adding prebiotic foods and probiotic supplements can help.

- **Quit smoking** – Smoking triggers inflammation.

Oxidative Stress

Oxidation is what happens to a piece of metal when it comes into contact with oxygen and water. When this happens, a chemical reaction occurs that produces hydrated iron oxide, commonly referred to as rust.

Oxidation in the body refers to the production of a "free radical," a molecule of oxygen produced during normal chemical reactions in the body. Poor diet, smoking, drinking alcohol, and chronic stress create an excessive number of free radicals. This can damage the cells of our body, leading to disease.

Oxidative stress is related to inflammation, but it damages the body in a different way. Whereas inflammation is a process during which the body creates chemicals as an immune response, oxidation is a process during which excessive free radicals damage the cells of the body.

The oxidative stress from an overload of free radicals contributes to aging. It also contributes to many other chronic illnesses including heart disease, diabetes, cancer, Alzheimer's, and Parkinson's. Excess free radicals also trigger the immune system, increasing inflammation.

We can also reduce oxidative stress by consuming antioxidant-rich foods such as fruits, vegetables, and nuts.

Dark Chocolate

Dark chocolate has a great reputation. It is loaded with antioxidants. Studies say the benefits of eating moderate amounts of dark chocolate, especially those containing 70% or more cocoa, are good for our health.

Dark chocolate is believed to reduce inflammation, improve heart and brain health, lower the risk of diabetes, regulate cholesterol, and protect skin from sun damage.

What's not to like about that?

The problem is that most dark chocolate we buy in grocery stores contain heavy metals, such as lead and cadmium. I learned this disturbing fact when I looked at the ingredients on the bars of dark chocolate I was eating every day. Not recognizing any of the words printed on the list of ingredients, I went to Google for information.

In 2022, Consumer Reports tested 28 bars of dark chocolate and found that some brands exceeded California's allowable maximum levels. Class-action suits have been filed against the makers of some dark chocolate brands.

I now buy organic dark chocolate because I don't want to poison myself with lead. I may be over reacting, but the following story demonstrates how long-term use of toxic substances may lead to problems.

The Downfall of the Roman Empire

The Romans used lead in everything, including their plumbing. In fact, the word plumbing comes from the Latin word *plumbum,* which means lead. They also cooked with lead pots and pans and sweetened their wine by boiling grape leaves in lead vessels, which probably leached lead into their wine.

The decline of the Roman Empire had many contributing factors, including economic instability, political corruption, plagues, and climate change. Some historians believe lead poisoning may have caused infertility, cognitive decline, aggressive behavior, and poor decision-making, which contributed to the decline.

No one knows if lead poisoning was a factor in the fall of the Roman Empire, but it raises the question of how toxins in our environment today may affect future generations.

Chapter Twenty-Two

A Pill for Every ill

Homeostasis is our body's amazing ability to stay healthy by maintaining the functions of our body regardless of external conditions.

When homeostasis is disrupted, chronic diseases can develop. Medications can be prescribed to treat symptoms of:

- High blood pressure

- High blood sugar

- Conditions related to the nervous system

- Breathing problems

- Infections

Medications are needed to treat illness, but care needs to be taken to avoid taking too many. Drug interactions can cause problems and drugs have side effects, leading to a cascading effect of more drugs being prescribed.

Many people are aware of the dangers of taking too many drugs. They take the minimum number of medications needed to manage the symptoms of their illness. Others are influenced by television commercials and want more.

Ask Your Doctor

The U.S. and New Zealand are the only countries that allow drugs to be advertised with television commercials.

The first prescription drug commercial in the U.S. aired in 1983, advertising Rufin, a pain reliever manufactured by Boots pharmaceuticals. The FDA pulled the ad, establishing their authority, and making rules drug companies needed to follow. According to Dr. Robert Schmerling, a Harvard Health senior editor, the FDA eased restrictions in 1997, allowing pharmaceutical companies to market their drugs directly to the public. This led to the creation of an estimated $14 billion-a-year pharmaceutical advertising industry.

Pharmaceutical companies spend billions of dollars each year creating commercials that show what a happy, healthy human you could be if you took their drugs. They include a suggestion to "Ask your doctor if this drug is right for you." Some are more direct: "Tell your doctor you want to try this drug."

A medical doctor told me recently that their practice has changed significantly over the past 20 years.

"Patients come in demanding certain drugs, and they get angry if I don't think it's something they need."

The FDA does not pre-approve TV ads for drugs, but they do monitor them. They can issue warnings or pull the ads if certain requirements are not met. One requirement, called the "Major Statement," requires a warning regarding side effects. The side effects are mentioned by a fast-talking voice at the end of the commercial, but the warning is overshadowed by the smiling faces and benefits advertised in the commercials.

Polypharmacy

"Polypharmacy" is a term used to describe patients who take five or more prescription medications which lead to adverse drug reactions (ADR). The CDC estimates that about a third of Americans in their 60s and 70s fall into this category.

Medications for certain conditions are necessary, but side effects and drug interactions lead to problems, especially in the elderly, including:

- Falls

- Confusion

- Dizziness

- Constipation

- Kidney and Liver damage

I've had elderly patients visit my office with lists of 10 different medications — sometimes more — prescribed by different specialists. One patient presented a list of 23 medications taken daily, plus several more taken "as needed." Some say they have taken many of them for years, sometimes decades. And some don't understand why they are taking so many medications!

Adverse drug reactions can be deadly. According to a 1998 study published in the *Journal of the American Medical Association* (JAMA), adverse drug reactions cause at least 100,000 deaths each year, making prescription drugs the fourth leading cause of death behind heart disease, cancer, and stroke. That was more than 20 years ago.

Research suggests that the majority of medical errors, including errors in prescribing, dispensing, or administering drugs are not reported, which probably makes the number of deaths per year due to prescription drugs even higher.

The American Society of Pharmacovigilance (ASP) says that adverse drug reactions cause 250,000 deaths annually and could be the third leading cause of death in the U.S.

Deprescribing – an Emerging Specialty?

Patients go to different doctors and different pharmacies, and sometimes, one doctor doesn't know what another has prescribed. Rarely does a doctor have time to research every drug a patient is taking to determine whether drug interactions are causing symptoms.

Pharmaceutical companies send sales people to medical offices to teach doctors how and when to prescribe medications — but do they offer support when it comes to deprescribing them?

It can be very dangerous to stop or reduce certain medications, and many factors need to be considered. Is the medication still needed? Can the dose be lowered? Are drug interactions causing problems? Do the risks of a medication outweigh the benefits? Some doctors don't have the training or time to ponder such questions and make these important decisions.

I recently heard a radio advertisement for a local medical clinic claiming they could help people make sense of all the drugs they are taking. I was driving and didn't write down the name of the clinic, and I couldn't find anything about it online — but it sparked a deep dive into the issue.

Many doctors, clinical pharmacists, and nurses are working together to find a way to address the problems associated with polypharmacy, especially in elderly patients.

A medical reference app called Epocrates, used primarily by health-care professionals, contains detailed information on thousands of prescription and over-the-counter medications. Information on interactions, adverse effects, and dosing can help manage medications patients are taking. Also included in Epocrates are clinical guidelines for managing diseases and tools for quickly calculating how much medication a patient may need based on their height and weight.

A company in Canada is doing research and creating plans for doctors to help patients discover if their medications are causing more problems than benefits. Their website, deprescribing.org, explains how they gather information and create algorithms to help doctors evaluate patients' medications.

Some studies suggest that AI will be useful in creating programs to help evaluate the need and risk-benefit ratio of taking multiple medications.

WARNING!

You should never change or stop taking prescription drugs without consulting your doctor. Stopping medication without proper medical supervision could be fatal.

Polypharmacy is not always bad. Sometimes, multiple medications are needed to treat different conditions. But sometimes, too many medications make things worse. Deprescribing is an emerging field of medicine. Challenges include the need to review prescribed medications, identify problems associated with dose or need, and develop and monitor plans to deprescribe if indicated. Doctors, pharmacists, and other health-care professionals are working on ways to meet these challenges.

Hope is on the horizon, but the question remains. How did our health-care system become a Sickness Care System?

Chapter Twenty-Three
The Flexner Report

In the early 1900s, medical education in the United States lacked consistency. Many medical schools lacked standardized curricula. In response, the newly formed American Medical Association (AMA) partnered with the Carnegie Foundation to assess the training of medical doctors. A study was commissioned.

In 1910, Abraham Flexner, an education specialist, published the Flexner Report. The recommendations in his report led to the closure or merger of nearly half of all medical schools. According to Flexner's recommendations, bio-medical research and training for doctors was implemented.

Between 1910 and 1920, the Rockefeller General Education Board donated about $50 million to reform medical education, which is equivalent to about $1 billion today. The Carnegie Foundation also granted millions to help implement recommendations of the Flexner Report.

Until the Flexner Report, natural healing methods such as chiropractic, osteopathy, and naturopathy were competing with conventional medicine. After the Flexner report, many natural healing methods were replaced with pharmaceutical drugs for treating symptoms. Osteopaths were invited to join the AMA in 1969, but chiropractors managed to survive and thrive as an alternative to a pharmaceutical-based health care system. But there is danger ahead.

The curricula of chiropractic colleges have changed over the past few decades. With less focus on enhancing the natural healing power of the body and more focus on medical practices, the profession is divided.

Some chiropractors, known as *mixers,* want the legal right to prescribe drugs. They say this will help fill the shortage of general medical doctors. Other chiropractors, known as principled or *straight* chiropractors, warn the profession will be dissolved and absorbed into the AMA as were the osteopaths.

Future Trends - Integrative Medicine

The Natural Healing forces within us are the greatest force in getting well.

—Hippocrates, the Father of Medicine

The growing awareness of people seeking natural healing methods has led to the emerging field of integrative medicine, an approach to health-care that combines Western medical practices with complementary techniques.

Major medical centers such as Mayo Clinic, Duke University, and Johns Hopkins have established integrative medicine departments. The field of integrative medicine is growing, not with the goal of replacing conventional medicine, but by incorporating evidence-based practices that address physical, emotional, and environmental influences that affect health.

Integrative medicine involves combining traditional medical treatments with evidence-based complementary practices, such as chiropractic care. Mind-body therapies including hypnotherapy, mindfulness, and yoga are also being included. Rather than just treating symptoms of the disease with pharmaceutical drugs, integrative medicine addresses the body, mind, and spirit of the patient.

There are many different parts to the health-care puzzle and doing what is best for the patient should always be top priority. When medical doctors, chiropractors, physical therapists, and other complementary practitioners can work together in the best interests of the patient, our sickness-care system can begin to resemble true health-care.

The Flexner Report had a significant impact on health-care in the United States by contributing to the decline of many natural healing practices. After the report was published, medical schools that offered training in alternative methods were either closed or forced to align with the more conventional allopathic model of medicine. The result created a health-care system that prioritized pharmaceutical and surgical treatments, as opposed to natural healing methods.

Part III

Physical Stress

Physical stress shows up as muscle tension, fatigue, pain, and stiffness. It's the wear-and-tear placed on the body through poor posture, overwork, injuries, or lack of rest.

Physical stress can also result from emotional and chemical stress.

Emotional stress triggers the release of stress hormones that create inflammation, which in turn feeds physical stress, while chemical stress from toxins causes inflammation that adds to the physical burden.

This section explores strategies to lessen physical stress by improving movement, rest, and alignment to restore balance and support the body's natural ability to heal.

Chapter Twenty-Four

Inside Information

When it comes to reducing physical stress on the body, a good first step is having a basic understanding of our physical structure. This includes bones, joints, ligaments, muscles, and tendons.

Bones Make Joints

We have 206 bones in our skeletal system that form the framework of our body. The place where two bones meet is called a joint. Joints are held together by ligaments, which are bands of strong connective tissue. Ligaments maintain the integrity of the joint.

Ligaments as Springs

Ligaments connecting the bones of the body can be thought of as thick rubber bands or springs. They have a limited amount of give. Stretching exercises help maintain joint flexibility and can reduce the risk of injuries.

Improper lifting, trauma, or other forms of physical stress can stretch ligaments beyond their normal range of motion, causing injuries known as sprains. For instance, a sprained ankle is the result of stretching the ligaments that hold the bones of the lower leg beyond their normal range of motion. This can happen when twisting an ankle.

Ligaments connect the bones and muscles move the bones.

Muscles and Tendons

Muscles taper off at each end and become tendons that attach the muscle to a bone. When a muscle contracts, the tendon pulls on the bone, and the bone moves.

Tendons are strong and healthy when we are young, but as we age, they become more prone to injury. Working the muscle too hard, without giving the tendons time to rest, heal, and strengthen after heavy or repetitive use, can cause inflammation at the point where the tendon attaches to the bone. We call this tendinitis (*itis* means inflammation).

Overstretching a ligament can cause a sprain. Working a muscle too hard can cause a strain.

Our bones, ligaments, muscles, and tendons form the framework of our body. Understanding what they are, what they do, and how they work empowers us to lead a lifetime filled with movement and vitality.

Chapter Twenty-Five
Our "Back Bone"

The 26 bones of our spinal column protect the spinal cord and give structural support to the body. These bones are called vertebrae. Between the bones of the spinal column are cartilage discs.

Cartilage Discs

Cartilage discs are concentric circles of strong connective tissue with a soft gel-like interior called a nucleus. Discs function as shock absorbers for the body. They also provide space between the bones for nerves to exit the spinal cord.

Disc Problems

Abnormal stress on the skeletal system can cause discs between the bones of our spinal column to bulge or herniate. Protruding from between the bones, a herniated disc can put pressure on the nerve or spinal cord. This can interfere with the flow of life force from the brain to the body, causing pain, numbness, and other symptoms.

Discs need water to stay plump and healthy. They are the first parts of the body to suffer from a lack of water. They absorb water through a process called osmosis. If we don't take in enough water, they shrink, reducing the space between the bones and putting stress on the nerves that exit between them.

Hydration

Everyone is different and has different hydration requirements, but drinking water when we wake up is a good way to start the day. After exhaling moisture all night while sleeping, hydrating in the morning is good for our body. It kick-starts metabolism, flushes out toxins, and provides cartilage discs with the water they need.

Depending on factors such as weight, activity level, or dryness of the air, recommendations include dividing our weight by two and drinking that number of ounces of water each day. Another common recommendation is to drink eight cups of water each day. High water-content foods such as melons and vegetables count toward hydration. Caffeine and alcohol act as diuretics and can deplete water from the body.

One way to measure if you are drinking enough water is to make sure your urine is light yellow. Dark urine could indicate you are not drinking enough water.

Drinking too much water can flush out minerals, causing low sodium levels and other electrolyte imbalances.

Discussing your hydration needs with your health-care provider can help determine how much water your body needs.

Degenerative Disc Disease (DDD)

DDD is not really a disease. It is a common condition in which the cartilage discs between the bones of your spinal column gradually wear down over time. The term is used to describe age-related wear and tear on the discs. It's a natural part of the aging process, like wrinkles or gray hair. It can be caused by genetics, repetitive stress such as sitting or standing too much, or trauma.

With DDD the discs in the low back or neck become thinner and less flexible which can result in stiffness or pain. Some people with DDD have no symptoms while others have pain, tingling, numbness, or weakness.

Treatments focus on managing symptoms with physical therapy exercises which work to strengthen the core muscles which support the spinal column.

Sometimes, DDD includes foraminal stenosis which is a narrowing of the space between the bones of the spinal column where the spinal nerves extend out from the spinal cord.

Knowledge is Power

If you are suffering from low back pain, it is important to know what is causing the problem. The findings of an

Xray or MRI will determine the type physical therapy exercises that will help a specific condition.

Extension exercises (bending backward) are good for bulging discs, but would make symptoms from foraminal stenosis worse. Forward bending such as pulling knees to chest would be good for foraminal stenosis but make certain disk herniations more problematic.

Besides physical therapy exercises, weight management and proper lifting techniques are helpful. In some cases, medication or injections are needed, but surgery is considered to be a last resort.

DDD is often thought to be irreversible and many times, no symptoms are present and it does not get worse. For some people who have chronic low back pain, DDD sometimes progress to the point where the spine stabilizes and pain decreases. This happens when the disc becomes so thin that the bones of the spinal column fuse together as if the body performed the surgery itself.

Managing DDD involves:

- Limiting activities that put stress on the spinal column, including running, jumping, heavy lifting, or too much sitting

- Quit smoking

- Engage in regular physical exercise to maintain flexibility and strength, especially of core muscles surrounding the spinal column

- Be mindful of posture

- Lose excess weight

- Avoid inflammatory foods

- Stay hydrated

- Consider seeing a physical therapist for expert guidance

Arthritis

We think of bone as a hard, rock-like substance, but bone is a living tissue. Bones can change in accordance with the amount of stress placed upon them.

The ends of our 206 bones have a cartilage cap, which is lubricated by synovial fluid. In a healthy joint, the bones move smoothly against each other, but when physical stress causes bones to become fixated, they cannot move properly in relation to other bones. Stress on the ends of the bones causes inflammation of the cartilage. Long-standing fixations can lead to arthritis.

The word arthritis comes from *arth*, which means joint, and *itis*, which means inflammation. Another phrase used to describe the damage to a joint caused by arthritis is degenerative joint disease.

The Takeaway

Our spinal column supports our body and protects the spinal cord, which serves as the body's lifeline. Understanding how it works empowers you to maintain a healthy alignment, prevent injuries, and improve your well-being for life.

Chapter Twenty-Six

Low Back Pain

An ounce of prevention is worth a pound of cure.
— Benjamin Franklin

In the United States, about 1.6 million spinal surgeries are performed each year. About 600,000 of these are low back surgeries,

Back surgery in the United States can cost between $15,000 and $35,000, depending on the procedure, location, and surgeon. More complex surgeries, such as spinal fusion, can cost up to $100,000.

Low back pain is one of the leading causes of disability, but surgery does not always fix the problem — especially if it's psychogenic, that is, caused by emotional stress!

FBSS – Failed Back Surgery Syndrome

Successful back surgery is measured by improved function and reduced pain, but it does not guarantee that all symptoms will go away. Between 10-40 percent of people who have back surgery end up with FBSS.

Symptoms of FBBS include:

- Pain in the back or legs

- Muscle spasm

- Weakness

- Limited mobility

- Difficulty sleeping

- Anxiety and depression

Other Orthopedic Surgeries

Besides back surgeries, about 900,000 skeletal-system surgeries are performed in the United States each year, including:

- Knee replacements

- ACL reconstruction

- Hip replacements

- Shoulder replacements

- Arthroscopic procedures

There are times when orthopedic surgery is the only solution, but a better solution might be teaching people things they can do to prevent the need for surgery.

Goobie Doobie

Known as Goobie Doobie to his subscribers on YouTube, Dr. Goobie is a MIT-educated neurosurgeon who graduated from Duke University Medical School. At the age of 38, he quit practicing after 12 years. Doobie is his cute little dog who appears in almost all of his videos.

His 2024 YouTube video titled, *I Was An MIT-Educated Neurosurgeon, Now I'm Unemployed and Alone in the Mountains. How Did I Get Here?* has more than 17 million views. Dr. Goobie, whose true name was not revealed until a year later, said operating on patients made money for both himself and the hospital. But it left him with a moral dilemma because he knew that, for many of his patients, surgery was not the solution. He compared back surgery to putting new drywall into a house with a leaky roof. He said it was a temporary fix for underlying problems including emotional, chemical, and physical stress.

He's Not Alone

Dr. Goobie is not the only physician who is disillusioned with being a doctor in the U.S. health-care system. Other physicians have posted videos on YouTube sharing similar thoughts and feelings.

According to the American Medical Association (AMA), many physicians are choosing early retirement, and many young and mid-career physicians intend to leave their organizations within the next few years. In their 2021-2022 survey of physicians, 46 percent said they feel valued by their organization, and 18 percent said they did not. Forty percent said they had moderate interest in leaving their current organization.

One problem facing physicians is burnout, which is often attributed to the amount of time spent at a keyboard documenting patient cases. In an online video, one physician said, "I didn't go to medical school to spend hours each day typing on a keyboard."

The word *doctor* comes from the Latin word for teacher, but with the demands put on them by organizations, many doctors don't have time to teach their patients how to stay healthy.

The AMA Recovery Plan for America's Physicians includes helping doctors use technology — especially artificial intelligence (AI) — to help ease the burden of clerical requirements and "let doctors be doctors."

Some AI programs being developed record the entire encounter with the patient and create documentation. This will provide more time for valuable doctor-patient interaction. In the meantime, learning to do what we can do to reduce stress can help prevent health problems.

Chapter Twenty-Seven

Ergonomics

Ergonomics refers to keeping our bodies aligned as we perform our daily activities at work or home. Proper ergonomics reduces physical stress and helps prevent injuries.

Guidelines include taking short breaks every half hour to help reduce strain on muscles and joints. Maintaining awkward positions for too long can lead to bones of the skeletal system becoming fixated, which causes interference to the nerves exiting from between the bones.

Posture – Becoming Aware

Becoming aware of the proper alignment of our body as we go through our day is a good first step in reducing physical stress on our structural frame.

Take a moment to notice your body position right now.

- Are you sitting with your back straight and your feet on the floor with your knees just a bit higher than your hips?

- If needed, do you have a little box or a stool under your feet if needed to make sitting more comfortable by taking pressure off your lower back?

- If reading this on a computer, is your screen at eye level so that you don't have to bend your head forward?

When it comes to preventing problems with your skeletal system, the way you sit, stand, and the way your head is lined up with your body as you perform your daily activities are important considerations.

For good posture when standing, you should be able to draw an imaginary line through your ear, shoulder, hip, and ankle. Rather than sticking out your chest and pulling the shoulders back, an easier way to achieve a more natural and effective posture is to:

- Imagine a string coming down from the sky. Attach this imaginary string to your breastbone, your sternum. Then imagine yourself connected to the string like a puppet who has hitched its sternum to a star.

- Imagine the string is supporting all your weight. You don't have to try. All you have to do is observe your chest lifting up easily, and feel your spine aligning perfectly straight.

- Allow your shoulders to rest comfortably on your rib cage. Allow your shoulder blades to relax, as if you are letting them fall into your back pockets.

Allow the muscles in your neck and shoulders to relax and rest on your rib cage.

- Many people lead with their heads when they walk, causing a jutting forward head posture. When walking, imagine a string attached to your navel gently pulling you forward. Let the string lead you.

Sitting

Following are some tips to consider when sitting:

- Chairs should be adjusted so that feet are flat against the floor.

- The knees should be at a 90-degree angle.

- Allow two inches between the edge of the chair and the back of your knees.

- When you write or type, your forearms should be parallel to your desk. Use a higher chair and foot rest if needed.

- The computer screen should be at eye level.

- Consider a monitor screen to prevent headaches from the glare of light.

- Arrange your desk so that everything is within easy reach, and you don't have to stretch.

- The chair should have enough cushion.

Text Neck

Text neck is a term used to describe pain and discomfort in the neck that develops when using mobile phones and other devices which require us to bend our heads forward for long periods of time.

Our head weighs as much as a bowling ball. The seven bones in our neck are designed with a nice curve to support our head in an upright position. Good posture is important to prevent stress in our neck.

When bending your head forward, the natural curve in your neck is reversed, resulting in stress on the discs between the bones. Spending too much time bending the head forward reduces the space needed for the nerves to exit properly from between the bones. The bones in our neck can become fixated, irritating nerves exiting from between the bones and causing problems, including:

- Neck pain

- Headaches

- Postural distortions

- Numbness or tingling in arms and hands

- Muscle stiffness in the back, jaw, shoulders, and neck

- Balance problems

What You Can Do

- Hold your phone at eye level rather than in your lap or on a table or desk.

- Consider using a cellphone holder.

- Take frequent breaks and do some slow and gentle range-of-motion neck exercises to release tension.

Too Much Sitting

The phrase "Sitting is the new smoking" became popular after a researcher at the Mayo Clinic used the term to illustrate the health risks associated with a sedentary lifestyle. Although there is no scientific evidence comparing sitting and smoking, a sedentary lifestyle can have negative effects on our physical and mental health.

The World Health Organization (WHO) says inactivity is the fourth-leading factor of death for people around the world. The average adult spends nine hours sitting each day while the average senior citizen spends ten hours a day sitting.

Prolonged sitting or lying down has been linked to:

- Type II diabetes

- Poor heart health

- Weight gain (Those who sit a lot snack a lot!)

- Depression

- Some cancers

- Dementia

- Blood clots in the legs

Crossing Your Legs When Sitting

When sitting for a prolonged period of time, crossing your legs twists the spinal column and increases strain on the lower back and hips. It can tilt your pelvis, leading to an imbalance in the muscles affecting posture and the way you walk.

Crossing the legs can restrict blood flow to the lower legs, which increases stress on blood vessels, and leads to varicose veins or blood clots. Crossing the legs can also put pressure on the nerves around the knee, leading to numbness or tingling in the feet.

Other Tips to Consider

Proper distribution of weight can prevent unhealthy curving of the spinal column. Women should avoid carrying a heavy purse on one shoulder.

Men should avoid sitting on a thick wallet in their back pocket. This can act like a wedge, torquing the pelvis and resulting in low-back problems.

Chapter Twenty-Eight
Exercise

Regular physical exercise is one of the most important things you can do for your health. Being able to climb stairs, carry groceries, play with your grandchildren (and great-grandchildren!), and live an independent life for as long as possible are good reasons to create a program of regular exercise for yourself.

According to the Centers for Disease Control (CDC) some of the benefits of regular exercise, not necessarily in order of importance, include:

- Lowers anxiety and depression

- Improves quality of sleep

- Reduces blood pressure

- Reduces risk of heart attack and stroke

- Strengthens the heart

- Strengthens muscles and bones

- Increases mobility

- Improves balance, reduces the risk of falling

- Helps maintain a healthy weight

- Reduces the risk of developing dementia, including Alzheimer's

- Reduces risk of cancer

Wake-up Stretch Routine

One of the most important things we can do is to start our day with a wake-up stretch routine that can be done in five minutes or less. A little stretching is better than no stretching. As I tell my patients:

"Dogs and cats naturally stretch when they wake up, and we should too!"

The following routine is easy to do and should become a morning ritual. It can also be done in the evening, before bed. As I tell my patients:

"Stretching before bed undoes what life does to you during the day!"

When performing these stretches in bed, do them slowly, and remember to breathe.

1. The first step is to flex your feet and pull the toes and feet toward the head in a pumping motion. Do this five or ten times. This gets the blood flowing and stimulates the lymph system, which helps remove waste products from the blood.

2. Take a few deep breaths to get oxygen to the muscles. If you have to get up and use the toilet first, do that. But then lie back down and get some oxygen into the system. And wake up! Because today is going to be a good day! Think it! Feel it! Say it! And most importantly — believe it!

3. Pull your knees toward your chest. Hug them if you can. Hold them close while pushing the lower back into the bed for an extra stretch for the hip joints. And remember to breathe! Hold for ten seconds or more.

4. Straighten one leg at a time and gently pull it toward you, stretching the hamstring muscles on the back of the thigh. An advanced version of this is to put both legs into the air and pull them both toward you, giving the hamstrings a good stretch while pushing your lower back into the bed.

5. Next comes the windshield wipers. With knees bent and feet on the bed, keep knees together and lower both legs first to one side and then the other. Note: A patient told me he wasn't so sure about the windshield wipers. Turns out he was spreading his legs apart rather than keeping them together as he performed the exercise. I think some cars may have windshield wipers that move like that, but I recommend keeping knees together! Another variation of the windshield wipers is to place feet hip-width apart before going side to side.

6. Neck stretches, combined with positive affirmations in the morning, can help set a healthy tone for the day. Moving your head slowly and carefully as if saying yes, think or say, "Yes, today is going to be a good day."

7. Then, moving your head slowly and carefully side to side as if saying no, think or say, "No. No negative people or thoughts are going to interfere with me having a good day."

8. Then, slowly and carefully lower one ear toward the same-side shoulder, and then repeat to the other side, saying, "Maybe. Maybe something really good will happen today," because expecting good things to happen is a great way to start the day!

Warning

If you are suffering from neck or back pain, you should be evaluated by a healthcare provider before embarking on a new exercise program. This will ensure you are doing the proper exercises for your condition and not making matters worse.

Crepitus

Crepitus is a word used to describe the crackling, popping, or grating sensation or sound that is sometimes experienced when performing a morning stretch routine. It is commonly caused by gas bubbles being released from the fluid in the cartilage lining the ends of the bones.

Crepitus can also be a sign of wear and tear on the cartilage. Most of the time, crepitus is harmless and of no clinical significance. If crepitus is painful or accompanied by swelling or severe stiffness, you should be evaluated by your health-care provider.

A good way to prevent crepitus is to stay hydrated and stay active. Low-impact exercise such as stretching, walking, cycling, or swimming keeps the joints lubricated.

Flexibility

Maintaining the flexibility of our skeletal system can:

- Reduce stiffness

- Prevent arthritis

- Prevent injuries

- Improve blood flow to muscles

- Improve posture

- Help maintain the proper range of motion of the joints

- Improve balance

- Slow down age-related decline

If we lead a sedentary life and don't move our muscles enough, they can shorten and lose flexibility. Regular stretching keeps the muscles long and flexible, helping to prevent injuries.

Some research shows that stretching cold, stiff muscles before running or doing an intense workout can lead to injuries. Before a race or a strenuous workout, it's better to take a short walk to warm up. Gentle stretching when you wake up or before normal activities is helpful. For strenuous exercise sessions, save the stretching for after the work-out.

How Much Exercise Do We Need?

According to the CDC's second edition of the *Physical Activity Guidelines for Americans*, the average adult needs 150 minutes of moderate-intensity exercise each week. This comes out to 30 minutes a day, five days a week. Two of these five days should include exercise to strengthen muscles and improve balance.

Benefits of Walking

Walking helps build strength in the muscles, tendons, and ligaments of the hips, back, and buttocks. It also helps prevent stiffness that can lead to problems with the joints. Walking gets the heart pumping, improving blood circulation to the brain and body and helping carry toxins that need to be eliminated.

The cartilage discs between the bones benefit from the increased circulation, which is stimulated by body movement. Circulation helps deliver fluid to the discs, allowing them to retain their cushioning properties and protect the bones of the spinal column from stress.

Studies show that walking can help reduce pain and stiffness associated with arthritis and the aging process. Many studies show that walking can reduce emotional stress.

Walking just 10 to 15 minutes a day is enough to get started. Gradually increasing to 20, then 30 minutes, five days a week. This is ideal. Everyone is different, and depending on age, condition, and level of fitness, the amount of walking needed to be beneficial can vary. Some may need more than others to gain the same benefit.

All you need to get started is a good pair of comfortable walking shoes. Make sure the shoes fit properly.

Finding a safe place to walk, preferably outdoors, is another consideration. If you cannot walk outdoors, walking inside is also beneficial. For more information on walking indoors, search indoor walking exercise videos on YouTube where you will find information and inspiration.

10,000 Steps

The number 10,000 was part of a marketing campaign used by the Japanese company that invented the first digital pedometer. They called it *Manpo-kei*, which means 10,000-step meter in Japanese.

The idea of 10,000 steps became popular and has become a widely accepted standard for physical activity. Many people make getting 10,000 steps a day their goal. They use gadgets to count their steps, such as an app on their cell phone. However, there's no scientific research supporting the idea that 10,000 steps a day is best for everyone.

Building and Maintaining Muscle Strength

Sarcopenia is a condition of gradual muscle wasting and loss of strength caused by inactivity. Sarcopenia leads to weakness of the muscles and loss of function, but strength training at any age can help rebuild muscle strength.

We're never too old and it's never too late to introduce strength training into our daily routine. Research shows that older people who begin rebuilding their strength make faster improvements than younger people who exercise regularly.

The key is to begin gradually, perform the exercises slowly and correctly, and allow muscles to recover for a day or more between each session.

Exercises to strengthen muscles include:

- Body weight exercises

- Exercise bands

- Handheld weights

- Weight machines

Certified exercise instructors, physical therapists, and chiropractors have created YouTube videos which provide instruction free for the searching. For instance, I searched beginner exercise videos for seniors and hundreds of videos came up, including:

- A ten-minute indoor walking routine
- Senior beginning home workout routine
- At-home exercise program for seniors
- Beginning weight training for seniors
- Ten-minute low-impact exercise for seniors
- Seated exercise program for seniors
- Seated chair yoga

Some feature music from the 60s, 70s, and 80s to help make exercises fun. Some require no equipment except for two cans of food or two plastic water bottles to use as weights.

It's always best to have someone guide you when you are learning new exercises. Watching some of these videos can help you become familiar with the exercises that physical therapists and chiropractors often prescribe to maintain strength and flexibility. And they are much better to watch than watching the news!

Squatting

Strengthening the legs is important because when you walk, all your weight is on one leg at a time. Standing on one leg requires strength, and lack of strength can lead to losing our balance and falling.

Squatting is a good overall lower-body exercise. It strengthens the muscles that hold our body in an upright position. Squatting is something we do every time we sit down in a chair. It's an exercise that can be practiced by people of all levels of fitness. If you are a beginner, to get started:

- Sit in a chair with arm rests, stand up, (using arm rests if needed), and sit back down again. Repeat.

- A chair is a good way to start. If you feel weak, you can sit down and rest for a moment before starting again.

- As you progress and your legs get stronger, you can move away from the chair and use the kitchen counter for support.

- Again, there are many free YouTube videos available explaining and promoting the benefits of squatting.

Before beginning any exercise program, I recommend consulting with a health-care provider. Depending upon flexibility, strength, overall health, fitness level, and physical limitations, there is inherent danger in performing strength training exercises. Not all exercises are suited for everyone. Injuries can happen.

Danger of Too Much Exercise

While most people don't get enough exercise, some overdo it. Signs of excessive exercise include fatigue, lowered immunity to colds and flu, and longer recovery time from overuse.

The Takeaway

Physical exercise is important for many reasons. It builds strength, endurance, balance, and flexibility. It increases circulation and helps eliminate toxins from the tissues and organs of the body. And it's your body's natural way of releasing tension and stress.

Chapter Twenty-Nine
Recovery after Exercise

Resting muscles after exercising is just as important as exercising them. Here's why.

When we exercise a muscle to build strength, we damage some of its muscle fibers. This is normal. Afterwards, the body begins repairing the muscle fiber. It is the rebuilding process that increases strength. For muscles to recover and grow stronger after exercise, they need protein and rest. Many people don't give their body what it needs to do this effectively.

Exercising a muscle too soon after a workout can lead to injuries. To avoid exercise from becoming counterproductive, proper rest and nutrition are vital between exercise sessions.

A Good Night's Sleep

A good night's sleep is one of the most important things you can do to help your body recover and heal, and should be a priority. Sleep can:

- Optimize cognitive abilities, including learning and memory

- Reduce emotional stress

- Improve our immune system, lowering the risk of illness

- Help maintain a healthy weight

- Lower the risk of motor vehicle crashes and other accidents due to lack of sleep

Tips for getting a good night's sleep include:

- Create a routine. Go to bed and wake up at the same time each day.

- Make sure your bedroom is dark, quiet, and cool.

- Exercise in the morning or afternoon, but not in the evening.

- Turn off electronic devices at least one hour before going to bed.

- Create a relaxing bedtime routine, such as reading and deep breathing.

- Avoid large meals late at night.

A good night's sleep is essential for brain health because when we sleep, our brain is able to eliminate metabolic toxins through the glymphatic system.

The Glymphatic System

Researchers at the University of Rochester Medical Center, led by Dr. Maiken Nedergaard, discovered the glymphatic system in 2012.

The brain uses more energy than any other organ in your body. Food becomes energy through chemical processes. This creates waste products that must be eliminated. It was found that during sleep, brain cells remove debris from mental activity by moving fluid through the brain.

Research indicates that the brain eliminates more toxic waste during sleep than when we are awake. This could prove to be important when it comes to toxic substances such as amyloids, which are believed to cause Alzheimer's disease.

Some sleep disorders require medical diagnosis and attention. Sleep disorders which should be discussed with your health-care provider include:

- Insomnia – difficulty falling asleep or staying asleep

- Restless Leg Syndrome – irresistible urge to move the legs, especially at night

- Narcolepsy – involuntary sleep that happens during the day

- Sleep Apnea – a sleep-related breathing disorder

Leave the Day Behind

As our day draws to a close and we prepare for sleep, we can use this time for meaningful reflection. Recalling good things we did during the day is a useful practice. Benjamin Franklin, often credited for this practice, said he ended each day by asking himself, "What good have I done today?"

He said this simple question helped him evaluate his actions and live a more meaningful life. It helped him look beyond ordinary tasks of the day and consider how what he said and did affected others.

Doing good is important, because recalling small acts of kindness and being helpful allows our body and mind to relax. It is during a state of relaxation that conscious thinking slows down and our subconscious mind becomes receptive.

Bedtime Prayers

Whether it's the Lord's Prayer, feeling grateful for blessings, or simply focusing on a word such as peace or love, ending our day with healing thoughts and words can improve the quality of our sleep.

Forgiving ourselves and others can be very healing. A simple Hawaiian prayer can be said silently as you drift off to sleep.

The Ho'oponopono Prayer

The following prayer is a traditional Hawaiian prayer for the purpose of forgiveness and reconciliation. It is used for healing emotional wounds. It can clear negative energy caused by the words and actions of yourself and others. It is a simple prayer, easy to remember:

I'm sorry,
Please forgive me,
Thank you.
I love you.

A Good Sleep Supplement

Deep relaxation is a powerful sleep supplement that helps fulfill our need for sleep. While it's not a substitute for sleep, 30 minutes of deep relaxation can benefit the body as much as several hours of light sleep.

When the body settles into a deeply relaxed state either through slow breathing or meditation, the brain waves slow down as they do when sleeping. Heart rate and blood pressure drops, muscles relax, and the nervous system shifts from fight-or-flight to rest-and-repair.

Rather than lying awake worrying about not falling asleep, gently reframe the moment. Use this quiet time to relax and let go, knowing that deep relaxation allows the body to rest, restore, and repair – just as sleep does. This is very helpful for those who can't always get 7-9 hours of recommended sleep.

Healing takes place during times of rest and recovery. When you give your body the rest and relaxation it needs, your nervous system shifts from alert to calm, allowing every cell to repair and renew.

Chapter Thirty
Preventing Injuries

One of the worst possible things you can do to your spine is bending, twisting, and exerting all at once. Examples include:

- Vacuuming or mopping the floor
- Raking leaves
- Sitting on a garden stool and reaching for and pulling weeds

We need to keep our bodies aligned with what we are doing. Avoid bending, reaching, twisting, and exerting by:

- Keeping the broom close to your body
- Keeping the vacuum in front of you
- Keeping the rake close to your body

Household Tasks

When deciding to paint a room, clean the gutters, trim a tree, or wax the car, take time to consider what you can do to prevent injury. Besides the basics, such as wearing needed protective eye covering, make sure you are physically able to do the job. Stretching and warming up muscles before starting any strenuous activity can prevent injuries.

Taking frequent breaks in the middle of a job relieves tension and stress and can help prevent injuries. A slight stretch backwards with hands on the lower back reduces stress on the spinal column.

Lifting

According to the Occupational Safety and Health Administration (OSHA), two million people injure their back each year. Half of those injuries happen at work.

Whether you are lifting a heavy item at work, at home, or in the gym, there are things to keep in mind so you do not injure your back.

First of all, never attempt to lift anything heavier than you can manage. Warming up before lifting by stretching and marching in place a few times can prevent injuries. Also, make sure you are hydrated, nourished, and not sleep-deprived. And plan ahead.

- Is the object too heavy or too large for you?

- Is it awkward, or will you be able to get a good grip?

- Is the area around you dry so you don't slip?

- Is the path you will carry the item clear?

Maintaining proper body mechanics can prevent injuries. When ready to lift the object:

- Stand close to the item.

- Bend your knees.

- Keep shoulders and hips facing the same direction.

- Keep your head up; don't look down.

- Squat down using your knees; don't bend forward.

- Never twist while lifting.

- Never lift an item higher than your shoulders.

- Don't hold your breath while lifting, carrying, or setting the load down.

- Hold the load close to your body at waist level.

- Avoid quick movements; move slowly when holding weight.

As you carry the item to the desired location:

- Don't twist your body.

- If you need to change directions, start with the hips turning and then follow with the feet.

- Take small steps.

Setting Heavy Things Down

- Move slowly; don't rush.

- Squat down using your knees and hips.

- Don't bend over.

- Tighten your abdominal muscles.

The Takeaway

Protecting your body and preventing injuries is not just about caution. It's about respecting yourself enough to move with intention while performing activities. Doing so will help you stay active longer so you can enjoy your life.

Chapter Thirty-One
Self-Care for Injuries – Ice or Heat?

When my car was hit from behind in an automobile accident decades ago, I didn't know what I know now. I used a heating pad on my back and shoulders, thinking I was doing something good for myself.

Using a heating pad on an injury is the worst thing we can do. Heat dilates the blood vessels, allows the clear part of the blood to seep into the injured tissue, increases swelling and inflammation, and makes the injury worse. Instead of a heating pad, I should have used ice, ten minutes each hour. Ice constricts blood vessels and reduces inflammation.

The next day, it was difficult for me to lift my head from the pillow. The next thing I knew, I was sitting in an orthopedic surgeon's office, being fitted for a neck brace. Wearing a neck brace after a whiplash injury is not a good idea, unless, of course, you have a broken bone or another serious injury that requires one.

Rather than immobilizing my neck, I should have been instructed to do small-range-of-motion exercises. Wearing a neck brace can result in an unorganized matrix being formed during the healing process. This can lead to adhesions and a permanently reduced range of motion.

No Heat for Injuries

When a patient calls to schedule an appointment after an injury, I ask if they are using ice or heat. Too many times, the reply is:

"Yes, I'm using a heating pad."

I tell them to stop using the heating pad and to use ice for ten minutes each hour a few times a day until they are able to see me. If they don't like ice, using nothing is better than using heat on an injury. When they arrive for their appointment, most patients say they are already feeling a little better after using ice instead of heat.

Professional Trainers

I've been to seminars led by trainers with a master's degree in sports physiology who work with professional athletes to keep them performing at their best.

One example that stands out was when a trainer shared a story about how professional athletes deal with injuries in real time. He described how a professional basketball player sprained his ankle during a tournament.

They kept him in the locker room all night, icing the injury 10 minutes at the top of every hour. They also iced the injured area for 5 minutes at the bottom of the hour. The body has a reflex and will dilate blood vessels in response to cold, but short periods of ice, 30 minutes apart, work well for acute injuries. The trainer said by the next day, it was as if the injury had never happened.

Alternating Ice and Heat

Recently, chiropractors, trainers, and physical therapists have changed their strategies. They say alternating ice and heat is better, because injured tissue needs blood flowing to bring oxygen and remove waste products from damaged tissue.

Following an injury, I recommend starting with short periods of ice for the first day or two. This will reduce inflammation by constricting the blood vessels and reduce fluid seeping into the injured area that causes pain, redness, and swelling. If the injury is healing, try adding a few minutes of heat after icing, then finish with ice and see how your body responds. Everyone is different, and different approaches work better for some than others.

Heat for Arthritis?

Applying short periods of heat increases blood flow to the tissue. This helps muscles relax. If the discomfort is due to arthritis, you can try applying heat for a few minutes to see if it helps — but use caution, as too much heat can increase inflammation.

Taking care of yourself after an injury is a powerful act of self-care that honors your body's potential to heal. Sometimes, self-care alone may not be enough. If chronic pain or severe postural distortions are affecting your life, you may need professional intervention.

Chapter Thirty-Two

What About Chiropractic?

The power that made the body heals the body.

—B.J. Palmer

According to a 2024 research letter published by the *Journal of the American Medical Association* (JAMA), the number of people using Complementary Health Approaches (CHA) is almost double what it was 20 years ago.

According to the report, the number of people in the US who received chiropractic care between 2002 and 2022 increased almost 47 percent. This equates to 37 million adults visiting a chiropractor each year.

Many people prefer drugs to treat symptoms because they do not understand what chiropractors do. They think all chiropractors "crack necks and backs."

Not true!

As a chiropractor with over 30 years of experience, I have adjusted thousands of patients without ever using manual manipulation. Instead, I use the Activator Method. That's not to say manual manipulation isn't effective. It's just a matter of personal preference.

When I explain to a new patient that I use a handheld, spring-loaded instrument to deliver a gentle tap for the adjustment rather than manual manipulation, some say they prefer manual adjustments. In those cases, I refer them to a chiropractor who uses manual adjusting techniques. Others are surprised and happy to learn that chiropractic adjustments made with an instrument also works.

Dr. Arlan Fuhr, founder and chairman of Activator Methods International and co-founder of the Activator adjusting instrument and Activator technique, has been generating a body of basic science and clinical research demonstrating the efficiency of the technique since 1986. In 2012, he was selected as the World Health Organization's delegate representing the World Federation of Chiropractic.

The Activator Method relies on reflex testing – specifically leg length analysis — to locate the bones of the skeletal system that are not moving properly in relation to the bone above and the bone below.

Chiropractic philosophy is based on facts including:

- The brain and nervous system control every function of the body.

- Reducing interference to the flow of mental impulses from the brain to the body helps the body heal naturally.

An Eye-Opening Experience

When I decided to become a chiropractor, I didn't know anything about the philosophy of chiropractic. All I knew was that chiropractic reduced stress on my nervous system, saved me from back surgery, and allowed my body to heal naturally, without drugs.

And because it worked for me, I knew it could work for others. After going back to college to get the pre-med classes I needed for admission, I arrived at Life Chiropractic College in Marietta, Georgia. On the first day of my new adventure, I made my way to the assembly hall with all the new students. It included a welcoming message from the president of the college, Dr. Sid Williams.

Dr. Sid, as he was known to students, was inspired to become a chiropractor after receiving help from a chiropractor in Atlanta for injuries he suffered while playing football for Georgia Tech. As I would later discover, almost every chiropractor and every chiropractic student had a similar story of being helped by a chiropractor who inspired them to become one.

Dr. Sid

Not knowing what to expect, but full of enthusiasm, I took a seat in the front row of the assembly hall, ready to take notes. When Dr. Sid Williams was introduced and walked onto the stage and began speaking, my eyes opened wide.

He welcomed the new class with an over-the-top level of enthusiasm that evoked a feeling of awe in me – a feeling I remember vividly to this day. He seemed larger than life. His booming voice, filled with energy and emotion, said that becoming a chiropractor was going to be the best decision we ever made. He believed becoming a chiropractor was answering a call from God to save humanity from needless pain and suffering.

I felt as if he were preaching, and I was hanging onto every word. He spoke about the body's ability to heal when interference to healing is removed through a chiropractic adjustment. I vividly remember his booming voice, declaring:

"Chiropractic First! Drugs Second! Surgery Last!"

I left that first assembly in a state of shock and awe, but in the coming weeks, months, and years, I attended Dr. Sid's lecture every Friday morning and listened to every word he said.

Maybe it was the journalist in me, but I saw this as a compelling story, rich with powerful quotes and stories about how the AMA launched aggressive attacks in an effort to eliminate competition from the chiropractic profession.

In November 1963, the AMA formed a committee on quackery. In 1964, they published their report in *Consumer Reports*, declaring chiropractic as quackery. The committee:

- Distributed anti-chiropractic propaganda to medical students and doctors

- Influenced newspaper columns and popular magazines

- Attempted to prevent chiropractic from being included in Medicare

- Made it unethical for medical doctors to refer patients to chiropractors

In 1975, a group of four chiropractors, led by Dr. Chester Wilk, filed an antitrust lawsuit against the AMA.

The judge ruled in favor of the chiropractors, and agreed that the AMA had worked for decades distributing misinformation and propaganda in their attempt to eliminate the chiropractic profession.

My Chiropractic Story

Before graduating from Life Chiropractic College in 1992, I was required to schedule an appointment with the financial-aid office. The purpose of this meeting was to find out the total amount owed on my student loans and to discuss my plans for the future.

When I told the counselor I was planning to move to Nashville and open my own office, she was skeptical.

"Why are you going there? Vanderbilt Medical School and Hospital is there and they are not very open to chiropractic."

When I told her that songwriting and music were my hobbies, she looked at me as if I were crazy, but I had a plan.

"I'm only going there for five years," I said.

At the age of 41, burdened with a massive student loan that would grow rapidly due to double-digit interest rates before I could begin paying it back, I headed to Nashville. I had one friend who lived there, and the phone number of a massage therapist, thanks to a mental-health counselor I had seen who gave me the boost needed for this adventure.

Knowing my background as a journalist, the counselor had some parting words before I packed my U-Haul and headed from Atlanta to Nashville.

"Maybe you can write a book about this."

Looking back, that's pretty funny, because here I am, 33 years later, writing a book about my experience of becoming a chiropractor in a medical-based health-care system.

Feel the Fear and do it Anyway

My first night in Nashville, I settled on the bed in the tiny garage apartment I'd rented in Green Hills, crying and praying to God for help.

The next day, I visited the self-help section of a local bookstore and came across a book by Susan Jeffers, PhD., titled, *Feel the Fear and Do It Anyway.*

Seeing the title of that book was just what I needed. Feeling the fear, I took a deep breath and went to meet the massage therapist who was willing to let me use her office on the days she wasn't there.

Because I use the Activator Method, all I needed was a massage table, my handheld spring-loaded adjusting instrument, file folders, and some business cards. This was before cell phones and computers. They had a receptionist in the lobby who answered calls for businesses like mine that didn't have a landline in their office.

Every time I went to the office, I stopped by the receptionist to see if I had any messages. Usually, I had messages from friends and family members calling to ask how I was surviving.

During the first week I had one patient, a friend from Fort Lauderdale — and the second week, I had two. As the interest on my student loan was compounding by the minute, I was surviving by going to the ATM every Friday and using my credit card to get cash advances to pay for necessities.

As a journalist, the morning newspaper and a cup of coffee were necessities. One morning, while reading the

Tennessean newspaper, I noticed the editorial page featured a daily 500-word column by a community member. That seemed like a great idea for me.

I wrote a story about chiropractic and delivered it to the newspaper. To my surprise and delight, they published it that week.

The receptionist at the office was overwhelmed with phone calls from people wanting to make an appointment to see me. She handed me stacks of pink phone message slips. Within a week, I had 30 new patients — many of whom had never seen a chiropractor before.

Here's the story as it appeared in the *Tennessean* newspaper.

"A Better Way to Heal"

By Dr. Fran Addeo

Chiropractic Physician

As a chiropractor, I believe the health-care crisis is the best thing since sliced bread. Because finally, after travelling the wrong road to health for too long, we realize it's time to turn around and try another.

When it comes to treating trauma and emergency cases, our medical profession is unsurpassed. But for most other ailments, the current approach of treating symptoms with drugs is the wrong approach.

Through their $1 billion-per-month advertising efforts, the pharmacological companies would like us to believe there is a magic pill or medication to solve all our health-care problems. But drugs are not the answer. The result of this erroneous concept is the current health-care crisis.

The word *crisis*, as defined by *Webster's* dictionary, is a turning point. So let's turn around. Rather than continuing on our path of drugs first, surgery second, and chiropractic as a last resort, it's time to try chiropractic first, drugs second, and surgery as a last resort.

Most people have no idea what chiropractors do. I, too, was ignorant during the two years following my car accident. I was under the care of an orthopedic surgeon who prescribed drug after drug in a fruitless attempt to cure my back pain. But because drugs are nothing more than poisonous chemicals, most of them just made me dizzy and nauseated.

When my doctor suggested I undergo back surgery, a friend suggested I see a chiropractor. Upon examination, the chiropractor explained how certain bones had misaligned during the accident, putting pressure on nerves and resulting in pain. And then with me lying face down on the adjusting table, the chiropractor adjusted the bones of my spinal column and neck. There was nothing unpleasant or uncomfortable about the adjustment – only relief from my long suffering.

I was so amazed at the results that I decided to become a chiropractor myself. Changing careers required two years of premedical studies before I could begin the almost four-year chiropractic program at Life Chiropractic College in Marietta, Ga.

Chiropractic philosophy is based on the fact that the brain and nervous system control every function of the body. The body has the ability to heal itself if it is free from nerve interference. This innate healing power of the body flows from the brain, down the spinal cord, and out to all parts of the body through nerves that exit between the movable bones of the spinal column.

It is the chiropractor's job to find and correct misalignments of the skeletal system that are causing nerve interference. When I adjust my patients, I explain that I am turning on the natural healing power of their bodies.

Most first-time chiropractic patients make their way into my office complaining of neck or back pain. Many are pleasantly surprised that as their misalignments are corrected, other symptoms, ranging from headaches to sinus problems to digestive problems, improve as well.

Chiropractic care improves the function of the entire body, although back pain is the niche that chiropractors have carved in their struggle for survival in a drug-based health-care system. (But that's another story.)

I began chiropractic college thinking chiropractors were back doctors. I graduated knowing the era of prescribing drugs to treat symptoms is drawing to a close. Someday, the practice of prescribing chemicals to treat symptoms will be looked upon as outrageous as prescribing blood-sucking leeches to remove pain-causing blood.

As we embark on a new path toward a more natural system of healing, chiropractic is a beacon of light shining brightly in our healthcare future.

Following the publication of that newspaper story, my practice was up and running, and I was busy helping others just as my chiropractor had helped me.

Helping Others

One of my first patients in Nashville was a pitcher on the Vanderbilt baseball team. His parents, who lived in another state, found me on the Activator Method website and sent their son to see me for a check-up. Nothing was really hurting him. He had some stiffness and soreness across his shoulders, symptoms most people would call normal.

Using the Activator Method of analysis, I found and adjusted segments of his spinal column that were not moving properly in relation to other bones.

He became a monthly-maintenance patient – not only did the stiffness in his shoulders and upper back disappear, but after getting adjusted, the speed of his fastball increased. He said his team had a device for measuring the speed of the ball and when his pitch slowed, he knew it was time to get another adjustment.

The Architect

Another one of my first patients was an architect who came to my office complaining of severe pain on the left side of his lower back. He said it hurt when he stood up after sitting in his chair. After performing an exam to make sure his case was a chiropractic problem, I suspected it was a fixation of his sacrum. I was correct.

His sacrum, located at the base of his spinal column, was causing nerve interference because it was not moving properly in relation to the other bones of the pelvis. Following the adjustment, he felt immediate relief, and by the next day he was completely pain-free.

This architect was an interesting case because the only adjustment he ever needed was an adjustment of the sacrum. He returned to my office a month later with the same pain, and once again, only one adjustment was needed. When he showed up again a month after that, I suspected there was more to the story.

I asked him about his daily activities and learned that his workstation required him to bend, twist, reach, and open a file cabinet next to his drafting table. Bingo! That was it! It was a simple case of bad ergonomics causing the problem. When he adjusted his work area, he no longer had any problems. I never saw him again, but during the time I was in Nashville, he referred several patients to me.

Bell's Palsy

A fifty-five-year-old woman who was diagnosed with Bell's Palsy came to my office with one side of her face drooping. She was told nothing could be done for her. She had never been to a chiropractor before, but feeling upset, unhappy, and desperate, she was willing to give it a try.

As she lay face down on the table, I used the Activator Method analysis, asking her to lift her face off the table while I checked her legs for a reflex. Sure enough, one leg pulled significantly short, indicating C5 was partly to blame. I adjusted C5, then checked and found that C1 — the very top bone under the opening in the skull where the brain gives rise to the spinal cord — also needed an adjustment.

The next day, she came into my office looking like a different person. Not only was her face not drooping, but she was smiling. She told me she was amazed at how quickly she began healing after the adjustments.

She said her family and a neighbor sat around the kitchen table, watching her face come back!

With happy tears in her eyes, she reached into her purse and handed me a small angel statue.

Dr. Sid was right. Becoming a chiropractor was one of the best decisions I've ever made.

Conclusion

A journey of a thousand miles begins with a single step.

—Lao Tzu

Managing stress is not an event. It is a personal journey that begins with a single step. From starting your day with morning stretches, eliminating ultra-processed foods, and taking the time for mindful breathing, you will begin to regulate your nervous system and awaken your inner power.

We all deserve to become the best version of ourselves that we can be, but we often expect too much too soon and judge ourselves harshly which leads to self-sabotage. Many of us were never taught to be tender and compassionate with ourselves, but that's exactly what we must do to move forward toward less stress and better health.

The journey to less stress and better health is a journey back to yourself – to the vibrant, peaceful, fully alive being you were always meant to be. The journey to a healthier lifestyle may have challenges, setbacks, delays, and disappointments. There may be times you get off track, but as Mark Twain said,

If you get stuck on the track, keep moving, because if you stay there, you might get run over by a train.

By using techniques in this book, getting back on track can be as easy as mindful breathing followed by a moment of stillness to reconnect to your inner wisdom.

This book is not just a guide. It's a reminder that you have the power within to steer yourself toward less stress and better health.

You have brains in your head. You have feet in your shoes. You can steer yourself in any direction you choose.
You're on your own, and you know what you know.
And you are the one who'll decide where to go.
—Dr. Suess

Let's Stay in Touch

Please go to my website **DrFranAddeo.com** and sign up for my newsletter to receive inspiration and more tips for having less stress and better health.

Acknowledgments

I am deeply grateful to all the teachers and authors whose wisdom contributed to my understanding of the concepts shared in this book.

Thanks also to Dr. Arlan Fuhr, Dr. Edwin Cordero, Sue Tompkins, Lisa Addeo, Dr. Phil VanAllsburg, Nancy Wallace, David Smith, and Dan and Joanne Fisher.

Bibliography

Ortner, Nick. *The Tapping Solution,* Hay House, 2013

Olien, Darin. *Fatal Conveniences,* Harper Perennial, 2025

Tolle, Eckhart. *The Power of Now.* Novato, CA: New World Library, 1999

Singer, Michael. *The Untethered Soul* New Harbinger Publications/Noetic Books, 2007

Murphy, Dr. Joseph. *The Power of Your Subconscious Mind.* Englewood Cliffs, NJ: Prentice-Hall, Inc. 1963

Dispenza, Dr. Joe. *Breaking the Habit of Being Yourself.* Hay House, 2013

van der Kolk, Bessel. *The Body Keeps the Score.* Viking Press, 2014

Robbins, John. *Diet for a New America.* Tiburon, CA: H.J. Kramer, 1987

Lappe, Frances Moore. *Diet for a Small Planet*. New York: Ballantine, 1982

Zelm, Dr. Jerry *What Your Doctor Never Told You*. Back2Health, LLC, 2010

Mancini, Dr. Fabrizio. *The Power of Self-Healing*. Hay House, 2013

References

- **Mayo Clinic Staff. (n.d.).** Stress symptoms: Effects on your body and behavior. *Mayo Clinic.* https://www.mayoclinic.org/healthy-lifestyle/ stress-management/in-depth/stress-symptoms/ art-20050987

- **Harvard Health Publishing. (2018).** Understanding the stress response. *Harvard Medical School.* https://www.health.harvard.edu/staying-healthy/ understanding-the-stress-response

- **National Center for Complementary and Integrative Health (NCCIH). (2016).** Meditation: In depth. *National Institutes of Health.* https://www.nccih.nih.gov/health/meditation-in-depth

- **Breit, S., Kupferberg, A., Rogler, G., & Hasler, G. (2018).** Vagus nerve as modulator of the brain–gut axis in psychiatric and inflammatory disorders. *Frontiers in Psychiatry, 9,* 44. https://www.ncbi.nlm.nih.gov/pmc/articles/ PMC5859128/

- **U.S. Department of Agriculture & U.S. Department of Health and Human Services. (2020).** *Dietary guidelines for Americans, 2020–2025* (9th ed.). https://www. dietaryguidelines.gov/sites/default/files/2020-12/ Dietary_Guidelines_for_Americans_2020-2025.pdf

- **Dunford, E. K., & Popkin, B. M. (2017).** Ultra-processed food intake and obesity: What really matters for health—processing or nutrient content? *Current Obesity Reports, 6*(4), 420–431. https://www. ncbi.nlm.nih.gov/pmc/articles/PMC5787353/

- **Liguori, I., Russo, G., Curcio, F., et al. (2018).** Oxidative stress, aging, and diseases. *Clinical Interventions in Aging, 13*, 757–772. https://www.ncbi.nlm.nih.gov/pmc/articles/ PMC5946307/

- **International Agency for Research on Cancer (IARC). (2015).** Glyphosate. In *IARC monographs on the evaluation of carcinogenic risks to humans* (Vol. 112, pp. 321–412). https:// www.iarc.who.int/wp-content/uploads/2018/07/ MonographVolume112-1.pdf

- **Owen, N., Healy, G. N., Matthews, C. E., & Dunstan, D. W. (2010).** Sedentary behavior: Emerging evidence for a new health risk. *Mayo Clinic Proceedings, 85*(12), 1138–1141. https://www.ncbi.nlm.nih.gov/pmc/articles/ PMC3404815/

- **Centers for Disease Control and Prevention (CDC). (2022).** Physical activity basics. https://www.cdc.gov/physicalactivity/basics/index.htm

- **Centers for Disease Control and Prevention. (2024).** Benefits of physical activity. *Centers for Disease Control and Prevention.* https://www.cdc.gov/physical-activity-basics/benefits/index.html

- **University of Rochester Medical Center. (2024).** Cleaning up the aging brain. *University of Rochester Newscenter.* https://www.rochester.edu/newscenter/cleaning-up-the-aging-brain-616872/

- **Psychology Today. (2025).** The medical monopoly on mental health and the Flexner Report. *Psychology Today.* https://www.psychologytoday.com/us/blog/the-leading-edge/202502/the-medical-monopoly-on-mental-health-and-the-flexner-report

- **Zollman, C., & Vickers, A. (1999).** ABC of complementary medicine: What is integrative medicine? *BMJ, 319*(7211), 693–696. https://doi.org/10.1136/bmj.319.7211.693

- **Cascio, C. N., O'Donnell, M. B., Tinney, F. J., Lieberman, M. D., & Taylor, S. E. (2016).** Self-affirmation activates brain systems associated with self-related processing and reward and is reinforced by future orientation. *Social Cognitive and*

Affective Neuroscience. https://www.ncbi.nlm.nih.gov/pmc/articles/PMC4814782/

- **Balban, M. Y., Hendler, R., Sun, J., Mahoney, M., Vago, D. R., & Huberman, A. D. (2023).** Brief structured respiration practices enhance mood and reduce physiological arousal. *Cell Reports Medicine, 4*(1), 101095. https://www.ncbi.nlm.nih.gov/pmc/articles/PMC9873947/

- **Keng, S. L., Smoski, M. J., & Robins, C. J. (2011).** Effects of mindfulness on psychological health: A review of empirical studies. *Clinical Psychology Review, 31*(6), 1041–1056. https://www.ncbi.nlm.nih.gov/pmc/articles/PMC3679190/

- **Gotter, A. (2025).** Box breathing: How to, benefits, and tips. *Healthline.* https://www.healthline.com/health/copd/box-breathing/

- **Wang, Y., & Qian, H. (2021).** Phthalates and their impacts on human health. *Healthcare (Basel), 9*(5), 603. https://doi.org/10.3390/healthcare9050603